FAT PIG DIET

WITH CARTOONS BY THE AUTHOR

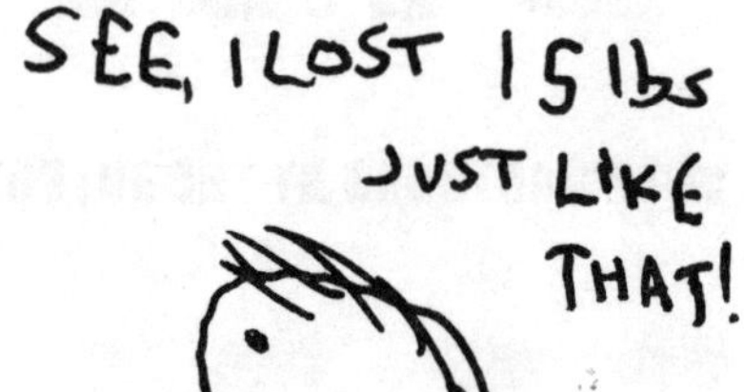
SEE, I LOST 15 lbs
JUST LIKE
THAT!

MICHAEL WINNER'S

FAT PIG DIET

BOOKS

The photo gracing the front cover of this book has been the subject of some dispute. I sat gracefully in a chair in my living room, whereupon a number of similar pictures were taken, some by Geraldine, some by my assistant Dinah. There was no way of knowing, for sure, who took the one that is displayed. I wouldn't say a row broke out concerning authorship of the photo, but when you see two virile ladies locked in mortal combat, which even went as far as fisticuffs and name-calling, it's just possible it could be registered as an official dispute. The front cover photo is hereby attributed to Geraldine Lynton-Edwards or Dinah May.

First published in Great Britain in 2007 by JR Books,
10 Greenland Street, London NW1 0ND
www.jrbooks.com

A catalogue record for this book is available from the British Library.

ISBN 978 1 906217 31 0

1 3 5 7 9 10 8 6 4 2

Printed in Great Britain by MPG Books, Bodmin, Cornwall

Always seek medical advice before beginning any kind of new dietary regime. The advice contained herein should not be used as a substitute for the advice of a qualified health practitioner. Neither the publisher nor the author can be held responsible for adverse reactions, damage or injury resulting from the use of the content of this book.

Contents

Foreword

This book is dedicated to me, to acknowledge my extraordinary talent and discipline in losing three and half stone (at times more!) and keeping it off. If you read these pages with care and dedication, and follow my exemplary lead, this joy can also be yours. If you don't you'll just remain a fat slob. This book is also dedicated to Geraldine Lynton-Edwards, a lady of astonishing beauty and, above all, character. You know the full quality of a person when he or she faces a crisis. At the beginning of 2007 I suddenly became crippled. It took months of hospitalisation and nursing care to get me back. Throughout that time Geraldine was more than a rock. She was a beacon and a saviour. At times of greatest travail she always presented inspiring optimism – not every time borne out by what later occurred! I always said, 'You live in cloud cuckoo land!' She is also possessed of magical powers, because after knowing her for more decades than I care to mention (she, dammit, gives the real number all the time!) we became engaged. I said at the time, 'It's taken me 71 years to get engaged. Don't hold your breath for the wedding.'

Let us be absolutely clear on one thing: the fact that I became ill at the beginning of 2007 did not in any way affect my weight loss. Prior to January 1st 2007 I had lost over three and a half stone and kept it off. With the illness I went down to eleven stone! But I soon started to put it on again. And because I was unable to do the exercise that I used to do before, dieting became even more important. I therefore brought into play the brilliance and genius of my Fat Pig Diet and have kept my weight around twelve stone, which is over three a a half stone less than I used to be in my fatty days.

Characters, not in order of appearance

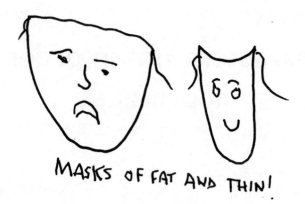

MASKS OF FAT AND THIN!

The outstanding photographer to whom ISM
daily reported his progress .... **Terry O'Neill**

ISM's gardener, who is nothing to do with this
book at all but wanted his name mentioned .... **Matthew Houston,**

and

As the couple who offered the most tempting
food to ISM, almost breaking his resolve to
stay slim .... **Sir Michael and
Lady Shakira Caine**

Our story is set in the present. There will be a 21-minute interval after
page 168 when drinks (in moderation) and refreshments may be
taken in the bar areas. Try to avoid crisps, nuts, ice cream and sweets.
No photography is permitted. Please see that all mobile phones are
switched off.

AND NOW, THE INCREDIBLE SHRINKING MAN!

Chapter One

From small beginnings comes a smaller Winner

Let's get the facts. For years I weighed 15 stone 10 pounds or 99.66 kilograms. On bad days, more. I looked horrific. I saw this fat, stupid face staring at me from the mirror. I was powerless to do anything about it, or so I thought. Then in June 2002 an ex-girlfriend, Geraldine Lynton-Edwards, came from Paris to live with me. A reunion! She immediately put me on a fierce exercise regime. Well, not that fierce! I did half an hour of Pilates every morning. Geraldine had been a famous and successful dancer and actress. She had been teaching Pilates in Paris, where she was living. Pilates is basically a series of stretching and breathing exercises. It is not aerobic.

This was the first sign of my managing discipline regarding my health, other than when I gave up cigars in 1994. Although Geraldine and I briefly split up, I still carried on doing 20 minutes of Pilates every morning, faithfully. This was remarkable. When she was with me Geraldine also made me walk an hour each evening. If I went too slowly she prodded me with an umbrella or a stick! I also somewhat curtailed my piggish eating. With the exercise I began to breathe better. I was somewhat more active. But I still got out of breath with a few stairs. I was still basically sluggish.

I notice a strange thing when looking at my diaries. In April 2004 I started recording my weight every day. On 25 April 2004 it was 15 stone. This was after some two years of just a little caution during which I had lost 10 pounds. But 10 pounds down in two years is not exactly a triumph, is it? On the last day of 2004 I weighed 14 stone 12½ pounds. Near as dammit still 15 stone! Then during 2005 I lost a stone by simply eating less and being careful. But I was still fat. On 31 December 2005 I weighed exactly 14 stone. At the end of 2006, only 12 months later, I weighed under 12 stone! Quite a difference! I was over three and a half stone down from my peak weight. All by watching what I ate. And eating less.

On the first day of 2007 I became ill with Vibrio Vulnificus, a little known but deadly illness, as a result of eating an oyster in Barbados. This oyster was not 'off' in the normal sense – Geraldine (we were by then reunited) ate from the same oyster serving and wasn't ill at all. The reason I got VV when Geraldine and other diners did not was because I suffered from a slightly fatty liver and had borderline diabetes. ('Three apples came up!' said my dermatologist.)

VV can come from eating an oyster from warm waters such as off Florida in the Gulf of Mexcio. It was only discovered in 1979. According to which statistics you read, up to 95 per cent of people who get VV are dead in the first two days! My dermatologist had never heard of Vibrio Vulnificus (he eventually learned about it by accident when lecturing in India), nor could we find any other British doctor who had. Nor had they heard of it in Barbados.

I was taken to hospital in Barbados and then flow by air ambulance to London. I was not expected to live. Indeed, I was close to death five times. If I did live nobody thought I'd still have two legs. Remember the old joke 'If you want to lose another 15 pounds cut your leg off!'? Well, that was very nearly me! An old joke with one leg! But I survived. One of the surgeons at the London Clinic held his forefinger a millimetre from his thumb. 'That's how close you were to dying, Mr Winner,' he said. 'Many times.' 'Then why didn't I die?' I asked. 'Because you didn't want to,' he replied.

Going back a bit… my big diet boost actually started in Barbados in January 2006. It was my irrational fear of dentists that put me on course to become the miracle dieter of the world. That's my view, anyway. I was at the Sandy Lane Hotel, a place where, normally, I put on a lot of weight. Marvellous buffet breakfast, suckling pig for lunch, great desserts. I'd had a temporary cap put on a tooth months earlier. It was sort of brass. My dentist, Nicholas Sturridge, who also does the Queen, said, 'Come back. That won't last more than eight weeks.' Four months later, I'd done nothing about it.

I flew to Barbados for Christmas and New Year. About 10 days from the end of my stay this brass cap became a bit loose. It was, as it were, coming away from my tooth at the top. Its sharp edge cut into my tongue. At first it didn't hurt much and then it hurt a great deal. Particularly when I ate. So I ate considerably less. I mean a lot less! I started to lose weight. I told my friend Philip Green (now Sir Philip), the brilliant retailer who was a fellow guest at the hotel, about what was happening. 'Pity it didn't happen earlier!' he exclaimed cheerfully. 'Then you might not have become such a fat bastard!' He has a way with words, does Philip. I went home and had the tooth fixed. But I'd managed to lose about five pounds in a couple of weeks.

Then I noticed something odd in my blood tests. Apparently the liver was not perfect. I went to see Professor Iain Murray-Lyon, the only person in the entire medical profession who never keeps you waiting. He said, after a few tests, 'You've got borderline diabetes.' He put me on a pill called Metformin. Some time later while having lunch at his house, Sir Michael Caine suddenly grabbed my hand and pricked my finger, drawing blood. He had a small, hand-held machine for testing diabetes. 'You haven't got diabetes,' Michael pronounced. I kept taking the Metformin anyway.

Three things happen when you take Metformin. You burp a lot. You fart a lot. And you lose some weight.

I went down another five pounds. I was getting excited. 'Sod this for a lark!' I thought. (That's the language I use when I think, 'I've lost 10 pounds. This could be my last chance. I'll lose some more!') But I was still grossly overweight. Whenever I went into the sea in Barbados, Piers Morgan, when editor of the *Daily Mirror*, would ask the paparazzi to get him the first photo of me emerging. He put it in his paper in a full colour page almost every year. The last one was captioned with a headline: 'What is large and pink and hangs from Michael Winner's swimming shorts? Answer, his stomach!' I was a joke fatty.

In this I am certainly not alone. Maybe you're one too! I'll give you an example. Stairs were a nightmare. I'd get out of breath. I'd have to stop halfway up. I'd huff and puff. I was pathetic. As I slimmed down and was helped in my breathing by Pilates, I noticed an astonishing difference. At one of my all-time favourite hotels, the Splendido in Portofino, there are some stone steps up from the pool to a landing. And then a further flight of tiled steps up to the hotel level. I'd guess 30 steps in all. In the past I always had to recuperate with a pause on the landing, then grit my teeth and walk up the last flight of tiled steps. When I'd get to the top I literally could not walk. I'd just stand gasping and wheezing. I'd collapse and sit on a window ledge. Then I dieted and did my Pilates. I climbed the same steps. As I reached the top a hotel staff member came running towards me with a chair. He wanted to help, bless him. But I wasn't out of breath at all. I just said 'Thank you' and walked past him.

At one of my equally top-of-the-list hotels, La Réserve de Beaulieu in the South of France, there are also steps up from the pool. About 12 steps take you to the garden courtyard. There I used to have to stop. Then I'd go up the steps to the lower bar area and another six to the lift area. By now I'd be leaning on the wall, totally out of breath. Same as the Splendido. After the Pilates and dieting I don't get out of breath at all. It's these regularly taken little journeys where you see, dramatically, the difference in what you've become from what you were. Surely it's worth dieting for that.

Please, take a suitcase. Fill it up. Put heavy things in it like books. Put it on your scales. I did this myself. I've lost at least 50 pounds. Feel the serious weight of 50 pounds when you carry it! It's horrific! You think, 'My God, it's not possible! I was carrying that around all the time in a mass of fat and flab! How did I do it?' Go on, please try this little experiment. If that doesn't convince you to eat less I don't know what will!

We hear a great deal about how overweight we British are. Fatter in the North than the South. Unhealthy anyway.

- In a recent survey 23 per cent of us were obese compared to 7.7 per cent of the Swiss. We are near the top of the European obese league (a newspaper headline: 'Overweight Britons among the fattest in Europe').
- The European Commission issued figures showing our average body mass was 25.4. Italy, the slimmest, checked in at 24.3. Malta had the largest number of fatties; their number was 26.6.

* A Department of Health survey announced that one-third of British males will be officially obese in 2010. By then one-fifth of children will be fat, putting them (with fat adults) at greater risk of heart disease, diabetes and cancer (it will cause 12,000 cancer cases a year by 2010, according to Cancer Research UK). To counter this it is intended to limit TV advertising of 'junk food' to children. A sillier government idea for 'tackling the growing obesity crisis' is in this headline: 'Overweight to get NHS dance classes'.
* A newspaper article headlined 'Epidemic of obesity could ruin economy' pointed out that healthy people remain longer in the workforce.
* A report by the London School of Hygiene and Tropical Medicine examined the link between health and wealth in rich countries and found that healthier people have higher earnings.
* In the summer for 2007 the Department of Health reported that people who were overweight became so because they ate too much. If that isn't a sign of total genius in the D of H, what is? Do they seriously think that people become over-weight by not eating at all? I can't believe some of the things I read about overweight people.

In any case, I no longer contribute to any of the disgrace-ful and shameful findings!

If you follow my diet you will not only be healthier but wealthier. You'll be saving Britain from economic collapse. You'll be helping us get to a lower position in the Premier League of overweight people. You'll be helping yourself stay cancer- and diabetes-free. What more incentive could you want? Let's face it, right now you may be fat, slothful, out of breath, heading for a heart attack – a perfect description of me from age 45 to 70. Before that I was overweight too but not as much. By the time I reached my sixties I was gross. Who wants to see a fat slob like that staring back at you from the mirror? I would turn away in horror.

I remember Jenny Seagrove, one day at lunch, in 1994, when I was at my worst, observing, 'You're blowing up like a balloon. Even your wrists are fat. It's very unattractive.' Later, Robin Morgan, editor of the *Sunday Times* magazine, was quoted in a newspaper saying, 'Only Michael Winner could make Brioni look like a sack of potatoes.' (In case you live on Mars, Brioni are the ultra-chic Italian clothes makers, whose items I frequently wear.) The trouble is, both Jenny and Robin were absolutely right. I was a blown-up, fat pig.

Of course I tried dieting. Many times. Even lost a lot of weight. But always put it on again. So how is it that at age 70 and two months things suddenly changed? What miracle took a man who could never resist temptation, who had failed at dieting for over 20 years, and changed him into a slimmer, healthier person? I shall tell you. You will do it too, believe me. If I can, you can. You will be healthier, feel better, look better, live longer. The only people who won't be happy will be your children. They'll have to wait longer for the inheritance.

Let's consider first why I didn't lose weight earlier – namely, I was a total pig. I was the sort of pig who'd have a salad in the kitchen, then walk to another room thinking, 'That's it, I'm on a diet. Done well. I've only had a salad.' Then half an hour later I'd think, 'I'll just watch the news on television in the kitchen.' Then I'd think. 'There's a carton of vanilla ice cream in the freezer. I'll have a tiny bit.' So I'd sit at the kitchen table, watch the news and eat the entire, previously unopened, carton of ice cream. I'd scrape the carton endlessly to be sure none was left. Then I'd go and do some work. Then I'd think, 'I'll just see if anything else has happened on the TV news.' Heaven forbid I should go and watch it in one of the six other rooms with a television. No, I had to go to the kitchen. There I'd find a carton of chocolate ice cream. I'd watch the news. I'd have a bit of ice cream. Then I'd put it away. Then I'd think, 'I'll just have a tiny bit more.' And I'd finish that carton off as well!

That was a typical evening in Winner-land. I bet you know people like that. Possibly you're one of them. As Oscar Wilde said, 'I can resist anything except temptation.' Or, as I used to say, 'I'm very good at dieting between meals.' So I'd try diet after diet. They were all ridiculous. And that's putting it kindly. They all had grand titles. On one they told you exactly what to eat every day, every detail of every meal. What a joke! You had soft-boiled egg and toast with no butter for breakfast. Lamb cutlet and broccoli for lunch. Fruit salad for dinner. I'm guessing at the detail, but you know the sort of thing. The organising of that, meal after meal, was impossible. If it got a result, the minute it was over I was back at the ice cream.

I considered liposuction. Or having my mouth wired shut. I wondered if I should go to a health farm. Then I thought, 'I couldn't bear to be with all those other people!' I desperately wanted to be thin and not ridiculous. But it never worked out that way. Occasionally a pill would come on the market. I tried them all. They gave me diarrhoea or other nasty results. With one so-called miracle slimming pill I put on six pounds in two weeks!

Then some nutty American lady fell in love with me. She'd been a check-in girl at Chicago airport. She made a fortune with *The Beverly Hills Diet*, a book that advised eating almost nothing but pineapple. Wherever I travelled I'd get off the plane and a chauffeur would arrive with a posh carrier bag of pineapples. I hate pineapple. The girl thought it was the way to my heart. Did she have a wrong number! Her diet proved to be vastly unhealthy. People all over the world were getting mouth ulcers. Being sick. They may or may not have been thinner, but what a price to pay! I was never on the diet, so I didn't care. There's another diet where you don't mix certain foods. I tried that for half an hour. Far too tedious. Far too difficult. And there's the one where you only eat protein. Your breath smells. Another absurd diet. I've never known anyone on it who doesn't put the weight back on afterwards.

I will now tell you in two words the secret of my diet, the secret of how I lost three and a half stone and kept it off. EAT LESS. I'll repeat that, because if you can manage this, it's all over, you're a thin, lovely person again. EAT LESS. End of story. Doesn't matter what you eat. Cake. Ice cream. Pasta. Who cares? Just eat less of it. When I decided to become thin I'd go to restaurants and only eat a third of what was on the plate. That was not easy at first. Worried restaurateurs would say, 'Is something wrong, Mr Winner?' I'd reply, 'Food's great. I'm on a diet!' If you set your mind to it, you can do it.

Another point (and this is vitally important): don't eat much in the evening. That's when there's no movement to help burn the calories away. You just eat, then sleep. You must, and I do mean must, keep food intake down in the evening. You can have an occasional blow-out, but cut down the next day. Severely. Also, weigh yourself every morning and every evening. When the pounds start to come off it's a terrific encouragement.

You know what's fattening. Bread, sugar, ice cream, pasta. Cut it down. Don't cut it out. My friend the photographer Terry O'Neill is a great dieter. Whenever we go out to lunch he orders two small starters. Occasionally he'll have a real main course. But not often.

You may well be saying, 'How much is less?' and 'How will I stand it?!' Well, if I, the pig of the western world, could stand it, you can. It's like when I had to give up cigars because I had a triple heart bypass and doctors told me, 'Stop smoking or you'll die.' I used to smoke 15 cigars a day. Did that for 35 years. Started at nine in the morning and finished at 10pm. By evening my voice was rasping and I could hardly breathe. Heavy smoke hung around everywhere. You would open my office door and hardly see me because layers of cigar smoke filled the room. People say, 'Cigars are all right, you don't inhale them!' Of course you do! I was getting emphysema. But still I went on. We all think we're infallible, that nothing will ever happen to us. After it did happen and I needed open heart surgery and a triple bypass, I cut down to two cigars a day until my final supply of 50 ran out. I had one at nine in the morning and another at 2.30pm or so after lunch. I got used to much less and then, without much difficulty, to none at all.

Thus it is with cutting down on food. You think it's impossible. But it isn't. It would be if you were forever denied some of your favourite tastes. But on my diet you are not. And then the most extraordinary thing happens. You don't feel ravenous in the evening. You don't feel an uncontrollable urge to pig out. As you see yourself looking better each day, as you feel fitter, you say, 'This is better than being a pig. I'll carry on.' Then you've arrived at a state of sanity. I never thought I'd get there. But I did. So, without any doubt at all, can you.

I was so desperate to lose weight I even let that marvellous hypnotist Paul McKenna hypnotise me. (I used to hypnotise people myself when a member of the Cambridge University Psychic Research Club. I was quite good at it.) I really wanted it to work with Paul. He kindly gave me a session in his mews house. I knew the routine. 'You are going to sleep. You are feeling drowsy. You can hear nothing but my voice…' Paul said. I thought, 'Just a moment. I can hear cars outside. I can hear a distant phone ringing. I can hear… Oh dear, it ain't working.' Paul carried on regardless. 'You are a little person standing by the door…' Maybe I nodded off, maybe I was hypnotised. But I soon heard him again. 'I'm going to wake you up now. I shall count ten backwards. When I get to one you'll wake up. You won't remember what I've said but you will lose weight.' He started counting. 'I'll have to do a bit of acting here!' I thought. He continued '… six, five, four, three, two, one.' I did a marvellous pretend wake-up. 'You were a very good subject,' said Paul. I wish I had been. I just went out and stuffed myself with food even more.

When you're fat you learn the tricks of not looking so fat. For example, wear enormous billowing shirts that hide your stomach, just as pregnant women have loose clothing. And never tuck the shirts in. If you tuck them in the bulge of stomach careening over waist and belt shows horribly. (I bet a lot of you are identifying with this.) Now I can actually tuck my shirts in and not fear looking ghastly. Another fat trick, when you're having a photo taken, is never stand in profile. Always face the camera. Then the stomach bulge doesn't show as much.

The greatest trick was taught to me by Orson Welles when I was directing him in 1966. He called me into his caravan one morning and said, 'Michael, you're not being fair to me.' I said, 'Oh dear, sir, I am sorry.' Orson, who became a dear friend, explained, 'You're always filming me from below. If you shoot from below it makes me look fat. I want the camera to be at eye level in future.' I loved and respected Orson, but you could film him from a helicopter and he'd still look fat. 'No problem, Orson,' I said. 'I'll have the camera at eye level.'

'Not your eye level,' roared Orson in that marvellous booming voice and with a twinkle in his eyes. 'My eye level!' Of course he didn't make me stick to this. But it's true. Every Hollywood cameraman knows that if you raise the camera you don't see the fat beneath the chin of the person you're photographing.

On one movie with Michael Caine and Roger Moore we were eating like crazy every lunchtime. Eventually when they looked at the stills they both said how fat they appeared. They'd put on weight. Matters were made worse because the stills photographer was very short. I did what any producer-director protecting his stars would do, something I've seen done in Hollywood many times. 'You'll have to stand on a box when you photograph our two leads,' I said to the stillsman. The stillsman didn't want to. So I had to let him go and replace him with a taller man! To this day I always tell cameramen, whether they're TV people doing a talking head in the garden, or press coming to photograph me, 'Keep the camera at eye level or I'm walking out!'

Now that I've lost three and a half stone it doesn't matter as much. But I keep doing it anyway. If it takes another pound off, good!

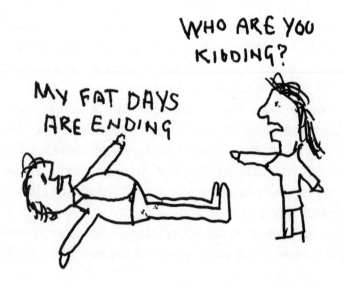

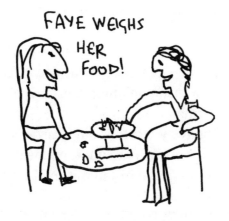

Chapter Two

Movie star slimmers whom I ignored

I witnessed the first very clear example of the 'Eat less' philosophy in 1994 when I directed Charlie Bronson in *Death Wish*. I'd been with him on two films before, one in Spain and one in Los Angeles. Although we dined together every day I'd never really noticed his eating habits. We'd always eat in a restaurant in our lunch hour. Charlie would spend the morning shooting muggers with spectacular accuracy. Then when we broke for lunch he'd leave his glasses in his dressing-room caravan and I'd have to read him the menu. He always left half of whatever he ordered. It's possible that as he was getting older, he watched his weight more. Or had to. When it came to dessert, which Charlie loved, he'd order one for two and we'd share it. I did lose a lot of weight on *Death Wish*. But I put it on with a vengeance when I didn't have Bronson guiding me. Just another failed attempt at dieting!

Faye Dunaway, to this day, carries a little scales with her whenever she goes out for a meal. And her own plate. She transfers the restaurant food to her plate and puts it on the scales. Then she scoops off food until the weight of plate with food is what she thinks it should be. Faye gave a dinner party in London not long ago. I recommended the Cipriani in Mayfair. 'Do you still take your scales along, Faye?' I asked. 'I certainly do,' she said. 'They all laugh at me, but I don't care.' I remember when Faye used to take salad in a plastic bag when we went out to dinner. She looks terrific to this day. It works. Don't knock it.

A great dieter, which may surprise you, was my friend Marlon Brando. When I first employed him in 1972 he started a big diet, even though, then, he wasn't that fat. He'd eat almost nothing but white turkey meat. I can see Marlon now, in my car as I drove to an Irish pub in Camden Town so he could meet Irish people and study their accents for his role in my movie. He was eating turkey meat from a Savoy Hotel napkin. He lost about 25 pounds but was still a tiny bit chubby when we started filming *The Nightcomers* near Cambridge. He took more off as shooting continued. Towards the end of filming Marlon rang me and said, 'I'd like to pay for a re-shoot of the first day. I'll pay everything.' 'What for, Marlon?' I asked. 'You were marvellous.' 'I was fatter then,' said Marlon. 'Forget it!' I responded. 'No one will notice.'

Of course there came a time when Marlon gave up dieting, although he'd always say to me on the phone, 'I've lost 30 pounds, Michael.' The next day I'd speak to one of his close pals: 'Marlon tells me he's lost 30 pounds.' 'Don't believe it,' the friend would reply. 'He's lost nothing. He looks just the same.' Pity, he was a dear and marvellous man. Slimmer, he'd probably still be alive.

Another dear friend who was endlessly on the most unsuccessful diets ever was Orson Welles. Every morning he'd have hot water and fresh lemon juice, which is indeed very good for you. Later during the day's filming I'd go into his caravan and find him sitting there bingeing on frankfurter sausages from a tin he'd somehow or other got hold of. He was like a child, was Orson. 'I don't know why the crew all laugh whenever they see me eating,' he'd say. 'They eat all day. Sandwiches, cakes, morning break, lunch break, tea break.' 'No one said life was fair, Orson,' I'd respond.

Inside every fat man there's a thin man trying to get out. Greed prevents him. My thin man was hidden below blobs of fat for 30 years. Now he's out and running. All right then, not running, but walking a lot faster than he used to. I was always the most undisciplined person in my private life. Now I am disciplined. It took me nearly 70 years. You can have a brain and do it earlier.

After lunch recently at a movie star's house I was telling a group of people how to lose weight. 'Eat less,' I said, 'and in particular eat very little in the evening. Also eat early.' A fat lady present looked at me with scorn. She was hoping for some miracle weight-loss diet to be divulged, the sort of utter rubbish that turns up on my email every day, often in triplicate, promising to make you thin. Nothing will make you thin other than cutting down how much you stuff in. This lady said, rather contemptuously, 'That's no good to me. I like to go out with my friends to dinner.' 'That's why you look like a fat cow,' I thought. That's why you're putting yourself at risk of cancer, which can attack fat ladies in particular, plus heart disease and many other delights.

Of course you can go out to dinner with friends. You have a Caesar salad to start, and at most a lamb cutlet with green veg to follow. And nothing else. Occasionally you can break out, which as you will see in my seven-month, day-by-day, dieting record, I not infrequently did. But basically you have to eat less and maintain eating less. Eventually those pangs of hunger that had me eating two cartons of ice cream after dinner really do disappear. Control, once exercised, becomes a habit. Even for pigs like me.

My friend Lord Glenconner, also known as Colin Tennant, the man who founded Mustique, once said to me, 'I don't eat dinner any more.' 'That's ridiculous!' I thought then. But he was right. If you're at home you don't need a big dinner, or anything more than a token dinner if you've eaten even a moderate lunch. So don't have it! Have the smallest snack as early as possible. Or, if you want to be really heroic, brilliant and clever, if you want to see years dropping off and people gasping in amazement at the New You, do as I do: have a glass of fresh vegetable or fruit juice and a water biscuit or matzo

– with butter and jam if you must. That's it. The pounds will run from you like rats from the *Titanic*. I eat 'dinner' no later than 6.30pm. Then I go for a walk, and then potter about. On nights I have to go out, I go out. I try to restrain myself. But even if I don't it doesn't matter much. I've lost so much weight that on the nights at home when I don't eat I can easily pull back any additional pounds.

This does not require you to be a superhuman capable of unbelievable willpower. I, a weak-willed moron, did it. So can you. You know what happens when it works. It's still happening to me now. I walk past a mirror and I see this thin person, having looked at a fat slob for years. And I say to myself (sometimes out loud), 'It's incredible. That's me! Unbelievable!' Don't tell me you wouldn't like to see a thinner you staring back from the mirror. Because those are the moments you can't hide. You see yourself for what you are. Better to see yourself younger-looking, thinner and healthier. That's for sure.

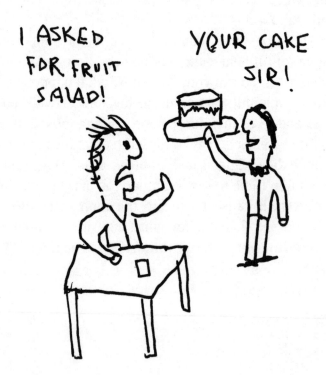

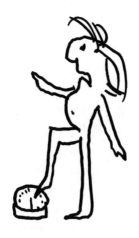

Chapter Three

The joy of the scales

This is it! This is what I want you to do. Next meal, whatever it may be after reading this paragraph, eat less. Much less to start off. If it's lunch forget the bread other than taking one mouthful to keep the taste alive, as it were. Forget the potatoes except for half a mouthful. Forget sugar. Forget dessert. If someone else has a dessert nick a tiny bit of it to keep you cheerful. Come dinner time, if you're at home just have fruit juice or green vegetables and a water biscuit. Before going to bed, if I feel desperately hungry, which surprisingly I seldom do, I'll have a mix of hot chocolate and Horlicks made mainly with water and a little milk. For breakfast I have sheep's milk yoghurt, with brown sugar to give it a bit of life, and clementine juice. You have something similar. Fruit. One piece of toast if you must. Now, you keep to this sort of ritual and you will soon see the difference. You will not faint. You will not be in agony. It is absolutely achievable. Later on I list what I ate, every detail of it, for seven months. Read it and note how much you can eat and still lose weight. During my diary you will see I started at 12 stone 12 pounds and ended at 12 stone. A further loss of 12 pounds. And that's after I'd lost, too slowly, two stone 12 pounds already!

Now, this is important. Never mind the idiots who say, 'Don't weigh yourself too much or you may get depressed!' Bollocks! Weigh yourself every morning. Stand naked on the scales. It won't be a pretty sight when you start. You'll probably pass or stand in front of the bathroom mirror and see a massive, ugly, protruding stomach, fat arms, fat face, fat legs, fat everything. But if you succeed, as I did, then you'll see a slim, younger-looking, different person. That is a real joy. That is an achievement you can be proud of. Weigh yourself before you eat anything. As soon as you get up. You may find something rather odd if you weigh yourself again after you brush your teeth and wash your face. The scales might show washing your teeth and your face has increased your weight by 0.2 kilograms, which is just under half a pound! Don't ask me how a few moments of doing nothing can cause that. But my scales frequently, though not always, show this has happened.

I always list whatever is the lowest weight in the first hour or so of waking up. (I need to be on the scales three times at that weight before I record it!) At night just before going to bed weigh yourself again, naked. In the morning you'll probably find you've lost at least two pounds while asleep overnight! Keep a note of these weights – a chart, as it were. It will soon cheer you up no end. It will be palpable evidence that you're getting lighter. Then, like me, you'll have to make extra holes in your belts and cut off the ends because they'll be too long. You'll either have to buy new jackets or have the existing ones taken in. Some of my jackets have been taken in six times, as I've lost more and more weight. You'll have to have your trousers taken in at waist and thighs. Eventually you'll have to have your shirts taken in both in the body and the sleeves. Or buy new ones. I've had two people taking in my shirts, all 198 of them. You see, if you succeed in losing over three and a half stone, as I did, you become a different person.

Reading my seven-month diary, you will see how much you can eat, which is a lot, and still stay thin or even lose more weight. I do not feel that I'm deprived. While what you eat for breakfast and lunch is not so vital, you can't be silly (you know perfectly well what 'silly' means). However, the key thing is dinner. I don't care how many times I repeat this: cut down on dinner and eat it as early as possible. At home eat very little. If you go out order less, order carefully and leave a lot on the plate. You don't have to stuff yourself until you can hardly move, then get up from the table exhausted. Burp and fart and go to bed. That was my pattern for years. I am reformed! I have seen the light! I can even see my you-know-what, which used to be hidden by a vast expanse of uncontrolled flab.

When you've come down to your target weight, you can eat more. But I found, even when eating a bit more, I was still in a cautious mood and my target weight kept getting undercut. It used to be between 12 stone two pounds and 12 stone five pounds. However, I was often three pounds under the lower figure. So when I got down to 11 stone 11 pounds, I thought, 'Now my target weight is 11 stone 11 pounds to 12 stone one pound. I normally only go out to dinner twice a week. But if I'm abroad I have some sort of more normal dinner every night. This will invariably put weight on, so as soon as I get home I'm super-cautious and take it off.

If, like me, you've had 60 or so jackets taken in, brought down another 40 from the attic, going back over 25 years, and no longer have any 'larger' size clothes hovering in case you put on, say, six pounds, then that's a real incentive to stay thin. Rory Bremner, whom I hadn't seen for a while, said to me at the dinner for Gordon Ramsay's 40th birthday, 'Where's your other half?' I thought Rory meant Geraldine. 'She's over there,' I said, pointing. 'No, the other half of you. You're half the size you used to be,' said Rory. It's things like that which keep you going.

I really don't want pitying looks from people saying, 'You've put a lot of weight on, haven't you?' Or 'I see the diet's gone by the board!' You grasp at anything that reinforces and encourages the effort to eat less and stay thin and even get thinner. Because although at 12 stone, which I frequently am these days, I'm three stone 10 pounds less than I used to be, I still have a visible stomach. It's just not hideously protrusive as it used to be. And I'm getting a bit gaunt at the neck. So it's either plastic surgery, or keep hovering around 12 stone. In respect of that I'm five foot nine or 1.75 metres. Used to be five nine and a half but it seems I'm shrinking in height as well as stomach. My ideal weight, medically speaking, is probably around 11 stone seven pounds. But my face would be looking very haggard by then.

So, now you're eating less, you're weighing yourself morning and night, and (hopefully) you're beginning to see results. Brag about it! Don't keep it a secret. When people say, 'You're looking so well,' you retort, 'That's because I've lost 10 pounds and I'm going to lose a lot more.' When they gasp, 'How on earth did you do it?' you don't have to say, 'Slavishly followed Winner's Fat Pig diet!' You can say, 'I did it all myself. I cut down on food. I eat much less. But I still eat all the things I like. Just not so much of them.' You will be a disciplined, sensible, healthier person. You may even shame some of your friends into following your example. If not, when they get a thrombosis and lie grunting in bed, you can visit them in the hospital and say cheerfully, 'Well, I warned you! You didn't listen to me. See what happens!' That'll cheer 'em up no end.

If you're faced with a normal main course – let's say roast beef, roast potatoes, gravy, Brussels sprouts, beans, with bread on the side – do you really think you'll go mad, be beset by neurosis, become terminally depressed, if you don't eat all of it? I used to bung down the lot. Now, unless it's one of my 'Who cares?' meals – and these are very occasional – I eat less. Half a roast potato, half the beef, one Brussels sprout, go mad on the beans.

Only a tiny bit of bread and butter. This way you still have a perfectly reasonable food intake. You can add a bit of smoked salmon to start and a nibble of dessert from someone else's plate too. You'll enjoy every single taste that you'd normally have, but you'll eat a lot less. Try it. Keep it up, and you too can be making new holes in your belts, getting new clothes or taking in old ones, and generally looking like a decent human being and not a bloated idiot.

I've lost over six inches around my waist. I used to struggle to get into a 44-inch-waisted trouser, often went up to 46. Now I slip easily into a 38. Mind you, I'm paying around £500 a week to my alterations tailor, who's still taking in (yet again!) clothes he took in only four months ago, and which he probably took in three or four times before that! Plus another substantial amount of cash goes out to two groups taking in my shirts. But it's a joy! I'm delighted. My cup – if not my plate – runneth over!

Please don't think, 'Winner's special – he managed to lose nearly four stone. I couldn't. I've tried and failed before.' I tried and failed many, many times. But when you get turned on to it, it really does become a way of life. And you realise, however piggy you were – and there was no bigger pig than me – that it does not involve great suffering. Concentrate the mind, I beg you. Don't just read this book and say, 'I can't.' You can. Try it. Eat less. Check your weight. See it going down. Your stomach will get smaller and eating less will become easier. It will always require some effort. But not nearly as much as, fat and slobby as you read this, you currently believe! Just say, 'If Winner can do it, I can. What's so special about him?' Well, I'm nearly four stone lighter. To me that's what's special.

I was a man who, for years, kept buying new clothes. I had to. I'd got too fat for the old ones. I bought new shirts, new jackets, new trousers. All bigger than before. And then I got too fat for those and I bought another lot. The old ones, the thinny-Winnie ones, went into plastic covers and hung in my attic. 'I may as well throw them out,' I'd think. 'I'll never need them again.' Now I'm wearing them. I'm wearing clothes made for me 25 years ago! People say, 'Have two wardrobes, a fat one and a thin one.' Bollocks! If I have a fat-clothes wardrobe standing by I'll certainly get fat again.

So don't think about it. Don't delay. Just start and enjoy the result. You'll surprise yourself. I amazed myself. I never thought (a) I'd diet, (b) I'd lose weight and (c) if I did I'd keep it off. I have and I'm not depressed. I don't feel stressed. I feel incredibly better! It won't kill you just to have fruit juice or vegetable juice for dinner if you're at home. You won't die if you go out and order very little in the evening. Yes, it does require willpower. I had no willpower for decades. Now I have. And I'm much happier, fitter, better-looking, more charming. People have said to me, 'If you were that fat why didn't you diet earlier?' I replied, 'Well, I still got the girls. Nobody reeled back in horror. So I didn't bother.' I only got going when, as I've explained, I lost a bit of weight in an unusual way and thought, 'This I will now continue.' If anyone had told me I'd be under 12 stone at the end of 2006, having been three stone 10 pounds heavier only a couple of years earlier, I would not have believed them. If anyone said to me I'd go from 13 stone nine and a quarter pounds on 1 January 2006 to 11 stone 12 pounds on 1 January 2007, I'd have said, 'I should be so lucky, but it won't happen!'

It is all possible. For you. For anyone. If you read the food-diary part of this book you can see it is achieved while eating ice cream, bread, butter, pasta, cakes, salted nuts, biscuits, cream and all the things other diets say you have to avoid. So take heart. You are not a lost cause. You are not a fat pig-slob irrevocably. You have a choice. I strongly advise you to take it in favour of health, mobility and happiness.

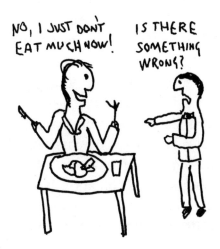

Chapter Four

A simple synopsis of how to lose weight

At first eat substantially less. You do not need three big meals a day. You certainly don't need snacks in between. Keep breakfast down to a minimum. A bit of fruit. Yoghurt. Coffee with no sugar and preferably no milk. Lunch, a little of what you fancy. Cut out, until you've lost quite a bit of weight, nearly all bread, potatoes, cakes, cream, sugar, pasta. Just have a little bit so you keep in touch with the tastes you have loved.

Dinner is the most important meal at which to keep intake down. When you start dieting just have fruit juice and water biscuits when at home. If you have to go out order a salad and another starter like smoked salmon. Chat away. Watch your friends pig out and look like pigs. That's their problem. They'll want you to fail. Don't let them discourage you. Keep alcohol down to a minimum.

Weigh yourself every morning and every night. You'll probably lose two pounds every night. See yourself going down. Like a lift. When you reach 'reasonable' weight – and you know what that is for you – keep dieting. From 15 stone 10 pounds I ended up at 11 stone 11 pounds! I did not suffer. On the way I even reached 11 stone 9 pounds.

Do some exercise. An hour's walk a day, even if it isn't fast and massively energetic, will help greatly. Try to do it in the evening. This will help you sleep as well. If there's a lift where you live or work, consider taking the stairs – not for 24 floors but, say, for up to three or four floors. This is what I did. Take it day by day.

All you need to do to lose weight is follow the above. You don't need stupid recipes that drive you mad. You can do it eating ordinary food in ordinary places. The simpler the better. You can't get it simpler than EAT LESS! If you're out, leave food on the plate. It's not a contest to see who can stuff more in, in the shortest time. If you're in, don't put food on the plate in any quantity at all. Just say, 'Today I'm absolutely not going to eat much.' Then see the result on your scales and be cheered – and say the same the following day. Once you get into the rhythm of it, it really isn't difficult. If I can do it – and I was weak-willed and stupid for decades when it came to food – then there's no question you can.

You will shortly be reading how I lost a further one stone and two pounds eating really quite lavishly. This is after already having lost three stone. I would never have believed I could have achieved this. It was beyond my wildest expectations. But I did and I'm alive to tell the story. Carry on reading. It could save your life.

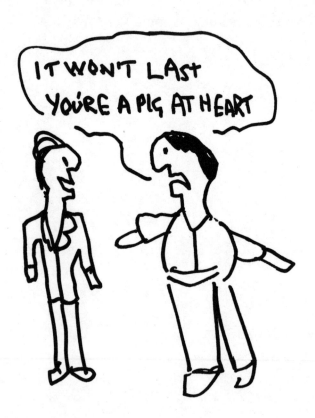

Chapter Five

You're slim and proud, but will it last?

You've lost your two, three or more stone. You're preening yourself. Luxuriating in the glowing remarks from friends, and even enemies, about how much better and younger you look. Now comes the tricky part. The part that matters most. You have to keep that weight off, or even reduce it. Not just for a few weeks. But forever. Otherwise, what was the point of losing it in the first place?

To help you in the main task dieters face, which is staying thin, I now present a day-by-day, night-by-night record of everything I ate for seven months. This will show you not just how I kept weight off, but how I further reduced it. Please note I start on 6 May at 12 stone 12 pounds. I end on 5 December at 11 stone 9 pounds. A loss of a further 14 pounds, or one stone! It's a roller-coaster ride in between. But it does prove that you can keep weight off, and even lose more, while eating many very substantial meals. And stuffing down things not normally associated with a diet, such as pasta, bread, butter, cakes, ice cream, potatoes and more stuff that's fattening.

I cannot repeat this enough: it doesn't matter what you eat, just eat less. In my diary I show you what 'eating less' means. You can see the daily battle we dieters fight to stay thin. You can also see what you can eat and what result it is likely to have. All this, very specifically. Torture it isn't! All it needs is reasonable vigilance, which you are perfectly capable of. Of course you're not going to follow this bite by bite. But you'll get a very clear idea of what you can eat and still stay thin. This is how it happened in real life, not in some dieter's imagination. Not noted from charts and theory. But in piggy-land curtailed. Along the way I've added a few personal observations about life!

SATURDAY 6 MAY
Morning weight, 9am before food, 81.7kg or 12st 12lbs. Breakfast: Delamere goat's milk yoghurt – two cartons of 125g each, one mini jar of Wilkinson strawberry jam, small glass of clementine juice. After breakfast weight 82.1kg. 11am: coffee from ground beans with Rachel's organic milk and big slosh of Bailey's Irish Cream, no

sugar. 1pm: lunch at Auberge du Lac, Brocket Hall, Welwyn, Herts, with Princess, aka Paola Lombard. Although it's not got much (nothing really!) to do with dieting, I feel a certain explanation of my convoluted private life is necessary. In the spring of 2005 Geraldine and I split up. (We'd actually got together and split many times over the decades before!) Shortly after, I had a fling with Paola. But we split up (as is my habit!) a few months later. Geraldine and I had stayed friends through the thin of thick and thin! Paola and I stayed friends too. (I remain friends with all my old girlfriends. This is because I am such a wonderful person.) The 30th of October 2005 was my 70th birthday. I was without an 'other half'! I flew some of my nearest and dearest to Venice. Geraldine was the lady I wanted with me for this catastrophic event. She was then living in Milan, working at her sister's dance school. When we met again I realised it was Geraldine, and no one else, for me! We even agreed to get engaged. But Geraldine didn't want to let her sister down. So it was not until July 2006 that she moved back to London. In order not to dine alone (something I've never managed to do!) I'd invite various friends to be with me. Thus it was – in case you've forgotten what I wrote a few lines earlier – that Paola accompanied me to Brocket Hall. The last time I was at Brocket Hall was with three of our greatest actors, all of whom starred in my film *The Wicked Lady* – John Gielgud, Alan Bates and Denholm Elliott, sadly now all gone to the great dining room in the sky. Then we had our film location caterers. This time I had three canapés: smoked salmon mousse in mini-croissant, smoked salmon mash on cucumber, and cheese straws in a dip. Starter of pan-seared smoked salmon, Jersey Royal and watercress salad, vanilla mayonnaise. Then pan-roast fillet of haddock with sautéed greens, brown shrimps and white wine cream, with mashed potatoes, spring carrots and green beans. A glass of Château Lamargue Costières de Nîmes 2004. Dessert, Grand Marnier parfait with chocolate tart and oranges in caramel. Evian water, two petits fours (one of chocolate-covered toffee and one sweet jelly-type thing), then real mint-leaf tea. Quite nice, Auberge du Lac. Lovely setting. Very good service. Food a bit bland but perfectly pleasant. It used to be 'run' by my least favourite chef (no, there are so many in that group it's not possible to pick the least favourite!), Jean-Christophe Novelli. Management said they fired him because he was never in the kitchen. The assistant restaurant manager, who was on duty, said he saw Novelli at most twice a week. Saturday he greeted guests in the evening. The owners should have written him a thank-you letter, because when he was in the kitchen the food was terrible. The *AA Guide* gave Auberge du Lac under Novelli two stars – a terrible rating. Next time the AA inspectors came he threw them out. What a twit! Now, having had four London restaurants close through lack of customer support, he's got his name on a ghastly pub in Harpenden, Herts. Thus are the insignificant fallen. 7pm dinner: one plate of fresh raspberries, three heaped teaspoonfuls of brown sugar, one 150g carton of Yeo Valley live yoghurt (contains organic milk), small amount of Malvern still mineral water. 8.35pm: bit of Rococo sugar- and dairy-free chocolate. Night weight 82.5kg.

SUNDAY 7 MAY

Morning weight 81.9kg or 12st 12½lbs. Breakfast: one carton Delamere live goat's milk yoghurt (125g) and one Woodlands live goat's milk yoghurt raspberry (125g) plus orange and clementine juice mixed. After breakfast 82.4kg. Mid-morning: coffee with Bailey's. Lunch at The Bird in Hand, Gosmore, Herts, with Paola. The reason I ate in Hertfordshire more than any sane person would is because Paola was desperately ill following breast cancer. Both breasts were removed and both ovaries, as well as further complications, and it was frequently too much for her to travel to London. At The Bird in Hand I had baked beans, chips, egg and sausage, bread, chocolate and vanilla ice, and treacle sponge. Still mineral water. A robust country pub, The Bird in Hand. Charming landlord, very pretty area. Don't have that sort of meal very often. Used to prepare it in the kitchen for myself, minus the chips, of course. But it's getting too much for me. To produce fried bread and grilled tomatoes and sausage and baked beans and fried eggs at the same time is equivalent to climbing Everest twice. A few years ago at Sandy Lane in Barbados, before they had the sense to have a marvellous buffet on New Year's Eve, as they do now, I asked them to do me a good old English breakfast fry-up at their grand New Year's Eve Dinner. At least it was fresh. Much better than waiting for staff, and a kitchen that can't cope, to serve 300 meals, most of them reheated. It was a great success. After lunch in

Gosmore we walked for one and a quarter hours in the countryside. I saw a fantastic, large oak tree root in a garden decoration place that was full of fake stone statues and gnomes. It was only £95 but I couldn't figure out how to get it to London. Dinner: strawberries with four heaped teaspoons brown sugar and 250g Woodlands live goat's milk yoghurt. Night weight 83kg.

MONDAY 8 MAY
Morning weight 82.1kg or 12st 13lbs. Breakfast: two cartons Delamere live goat's milk yoghurt (125g each) with a small pot of marmalade and clementine juice. Coffee at 11-ish with Bailey's Irish Cream, no sugar. Lunch: chilli con carne with rice, tortillas, crème fraîche, tomato, avocado, grated cheese, onions. Still mineral water. Mid-afternoon: iced coffee with organic milk and two heaped teaspoons of white granulated sugar. Dinner: salad with hard-boiled eggs, tomatoes, lettuce, salmon mousse, one piece of matzo with butter, one small chocolate biscuit. Still mineral water. After dinner one smallish piece of Rococo chocolate. Night weight 82.7kg.

TUESDAY 9 MAY
Morning weight 81.7kg or 12st 12lbs. Breakfast: two 125g Delamere live goat's milk yoghurts plus a mini jar of jam. Coffee 11-ish with Bailey's Irish Cream and milk. Lunch at The Ivy with presenter's agent Anne Sweetbaum. Anne is helping in the background with negotiations for a TV series, starring me, that may or may not happen! She was a prominent actress in the 1970s with enormous bosoms. I remember a picture of

her on display at the Globe Theatre in Shaftesbury
Avenue (now called the Gielgud Theatre), where she
had a leading role in *Play It Again, Sam* – one of those
images you don't forget. I had Buck's Fizz, a little piece
of bread and butter, Caesar salad with croûtons,
fishcake with extra sauce, cauliflower au gratin,
cabbage, rhubarb tart with clotted cream. Fresh mint-
leaf tea. Still mineral water. The Ivy maintains a
remarkable standard of comfort food, efficiently
presented. There's a pleasant atmosphere. It deserves
its place in the stratosphere. There was a chef sitting in
the bar area as I came out. 'Are you the chef?' I asked.
'One of them,' he replied. 'Congratulations anyway, to
all of you,' I said. And went out to face the paparazzi.
Dinner at 6.30pm: cold fresh crab and salad. Ribena.
Night weight 82.6kg.

WEDNESDAY 10 MAY
Morning weight 82.1kg or 12st 13lbs. Breakfast: two
125g Delamere live goat's milk yoghurts, one small jar
jam/marmalade and clementine juice. 10-ish: coffee
with Bailey's Irish Cream. Lunch at Petersham Nurseries
Café with theatre impresario Michael White. I met
Michael in 1963 when a man named William Donaldson,
who presented *Beyond the Fringe*, asked me to join him
in a theatrical venture called *Nights at the Comedy*. It
was to be a sort of variety show compered by Nicol
Williamson – who walked out a week before opening
night! Donaldson was co-producing with Michael White,
then a young theatre presenter. When the poster came
out it said, 'William Donaldson in association with

Michael Winner presents *Nights at the Comedy*.' I said, 'Willy, where's Michael White's name?' Donaldson replied, 'I've got you. I don't need him.' Thus Michael was knifed out! I was only in for £350. The show got rave reviews and was a disaster. The cast included Jimmy James and Jimmy Tarbuck. Donaldson, who we all thought was very wealthy and came from a rich shipping family, suddenly skipped town, leaving the cast and many other creditors unpaid. He simply vanished. The Royal Court Theatre, who'd provided the set, threatened to sue me personally if I didn't pay for it! Bloody cheek. I was just an investor. They withdrew. Michael White, who'd been cheated out of the show, paid the cast salaries for three weeks! Later he wrote in his autobiography – by then he'd put on *The Rocky Horror Show* and other successes – about how disappointed he was that Donaldson axed him from *Nights at the Comedy*. But he never said he paid the cast out of the kindness of his heart! I asked him why. He replied, 'Because I thought it would make me look silly.' There's an honourable man. Donaldson, who was posh and well spoken, was in fact a rogue. He vanished, leaving actors and suppliers unpaid, more than once. He became famous as an author and for running a brothel after he married a prostitute. He wrote about it in a brilliant book called *Both the Ladies and the Gentlemen*. Donaldson also wrote *The Henry Root Letters*, where he sent famous people strange letters and published their odd replies. He died a few years ago. At my lunch with Michael White, I ate a small amount of bread and butter, shaved raw asparagus with celery and anchovy vinaigrette, wild salmon with garlic shoots and sauce verte, warm orange and stem ginger pudding, French strawberries with crème anglais, home-made lemonade, crystallised rose petals with rose syrup tipped over and topped up with prosecco. The food at Petersham Nurseries Café is outstanding. The restaurant manager is the worst. Dinner: fresh raspberries with 450g of Rachel's organic luxury Greek-style bio yoghurt, brown granulated sugar and one mini pot raspberry jam. Mineral water. Night weight 82.4kg.

THURSDAY 11 MAY
Morning weight 82kg or 12st 12¾lbs. Breakfast: goat's milk yoghurt, jam and clementine juice. 11-ish: coffee with Bailey's Irish Cream and organic milk. Lunch: roast chicken, tiny bit of stuffing, one roast potato, sprouts, carrots. Mineral water. 4pm: iced coffee with Bailey's Irish Cream and organic milk. Dinner: roast chicken with tomato and lettuce salad, Hellmann's mayonnaise, two teaspoons of smooth peanut butter, still mineral water. Night weight 82.6kg.

FRIDAY 12 MAY
Morning weight 81.6kg or 12st 11¾lbs. Going down! This is very, very good. Breakfast: goat's milk yoghurt, jam, clementine juice. 10.30: coffee with Bailey's. 11am: piece of Rococo sugar- and dairy-free chocolate. Lunch: spaghetti bolognese with butter and Parmesan cheese, still mineral water. In the afternoon I had a meeting with people from Shine TV about this TV series where I go around restaurants and kind of review them. When I told

David Frost this show was in the air he said, 'It's got hit written all over it!' I said, 'Can I take that to the bank, David?' Dinner: grilled salmon and asparagus with hollandaise sauce. Night weight 82.3kg.

SATURDAY 13 MAY
Morning weight 81.6kg or 12st 11¾lbs. Breakfast: goat's milk yoghurt, jam, clementine juice. 10.30: coffee with Bailey's Irish Cream. Lunch at The Bull in Cottered, Herts: French onion soup with a cheese croûton plus a small amount of bread and butter. Hamburger on bun with mature Cheddar and bacon, some salad, new potatoes with butter added by me. Tastes of apple and raspberry crumble with custard, sticky date cake with toffee sauce and chocolate chip ice cream, bread and butter pudding with vanilla ice cream, and strawberries and crème anglais. A Pimms, still mineral water, fresh mint tea. The Bull is superior pub food. The desserts were amazing. This meal will do damage, even though I went for a walk afterwards in fields behind the pub. Dinner: 250g Woodlands live goat's milk yoghurt with raspberries and four heaped teaspoonfuls of brown granulated sugar. Night weight 82.9kg.

SUNDAY 14 MAY
Morning weight 82kg or 12st 12¾lbs. Breakfast: 180g St Helen's Farm bio goat's milk yoghurt with a pot of jam in it, orange and clementine juice. Lunch with Sir Michael and Lady Shakira Caine at their Surrey home: two Pimms, grilled salmon, various vegetables, new potatoes, still water, meringue with fruit and cream, mint tea without

milk or sugar, one chocolate-covered mint; later ordinary tea with milk, no sugar. Afterwards walked for about an hour with Shakira and other guests while Michael stayed home and watched cricket. In fact, he dozed off in a big armchair in front of the TV. So would I if I was watching cricket. I'd eaten a big lunch but balanced by a small dinner of 180g St Helen's Farm bio natural goat's milk yoghurt with strawberries, raspberries and brown sugar, still mineral water. Night weight 83.2kg.

MONDAY 15 MAY

Morning weight 82.1kg or 12st 13lbs. Breakfast: goat's milk yoghurt, jam, clementine juice. 11-ish: Coffee with Bailey's Irish Cream. Lunch: shrimps in a sauce, carrots, beans, rice. Still Malvern mineral water. Dinner at E&O in Notting Hill Gate at 7.30pm: some fruit smoothie with sugar in it, date and water chestnut gyozas, baby pork spare ribs, black cod with sweet miso, still mineral water. E&O is one of my favourite places. It has a canteen-like atmosphere, but everything is very tasty and the service is cheerful and exemplary. They even get a few glitterati. I've seen Patsy Kensit (twice!) and J K Rowling, who lives at the bottom of my road. My assistant Dinah said she saw Bono from U2 staring at me! However, this meal was dangerous. Too much. And even though we started eating at 7.30pm, too late! Night weight 83.5kg.

TUESDAY 16 MAY

Morning weight 82.9kg or 13st¾lb. A disaster! I've put on one and three-quarter pounds. I am getting close to the danger zone! This is what happens when you eat too much for dinner! Beware! Breakfast: goat's milk yoghurt, jam, clementine juice. 11-ish: coffee with Bailey's Irish Cream. Lunch: Lancashire hotpot with sliced potatoes, beans and carrots. Small portions of all! Still mineral water. 4pm-ish: coffee with Bailey's Irish Cream. Dinner 6.30pm: vegetable soup, two pieces of matzos with butter, still mineral water. Night weight 83.2kg.

WEDNESDAY 17 MAY
Morning weight 82.4kg or 12st 13¾lbs. See, hardly any dinner last night and I'm back below 13 stone again! Clever me! Breakfast: goat's milk yoghurt, jam, clementine juice. 11-ish: coffee with Bailey's Irish Cream. Lunch at Scalini, in Walton Street, Knightsbridge, with the adorable Koo Stark. Koo has the most beautifully behaved and charming nine-year-old daughter possible. I had two bowls of tomatoes cut up and in oil with a little bread while I waited for her. She was 20 minutes late. Naughty girl. I ate a grilled sole with fried zucchini and an espresso coffee. Scalini is one of the few places you can get a really good, juicy, not dried-up, large sole. The food and the service are beyond reproach. But it's too noisy. Koo is very interesting but it became difficult to hear what she was saying. Dinner: one small piece of grilled liver, a small amount of cauliflower and broccoli. Still mineral water. One small chocolate biscuit. Night weight 83.4kg.

THURSDAY 18 MAY
Morning weight 82.8kg or 13st ½lb. This is very depressing. I hate being anything over 13 stone. I don't understand it. I didn't eat much yesterday, did I? Maybe I

pigged out too much on the fried zucchini. The situation is even more dangerous because I have to eat at The Ivy tonight and my guests can't be there before 8.30. Otherwise I'd have them there at 6.30! We shall see! Breakfast: goat's milk yoghurt, jam, clementine juice. 10.30: coffee with Bailey's Irish Cream. Should've left out the Bailey's really, but I'm addicted. Lunch: fish pie with fresh peas and corn off the cob, still mineral water. 3.30pm: small piece sugar- and dairy-free Rococo chocolate. Dinner at The Ivy: Buck's Fizz (fresh orange juice and champagne), still mineral water, 50 grams Beluga caviar with blinis, Evesham English asparagus with hollandaise sauce, champagne jelly with cream, tea of fresh mint leaves and hot water. There was a slight sense of apprehension among the staff. Jeremy King and Chris Corbin had just nicked their long-time chief, Mitchell Everard – who'd worked at The Ivy for Chris and Jeremy before they sold it – to head their upcoming new restaurant in nearby Regent Street. The food and service were excellent as ever. But I was none too pleased with the way my reservation had been handled. I always fax The Ivy, asking for my usual table. Someone I didn't know, called Ben, phoned my PA and said, 'That's fine. I'll do my best to get Mr Winner his usual table.' That means nothing to me. I wasn't asking for someone to do their best. That's a weak 'maybe'. I asked for my usual table. That required a clear Yes or No answer. So now I had to phone myself. 'You've got your usual table,' said a nice lady. 'Then why didn't Ben say so?' I asked. 'He'll get a tiny mouthful from me when I turn up.' When I arrived that evening the staff were giggling. 'Ben nearly had a nervous breakdown,' they said. But Ben was not in sight. He'd been transferred to their sister restaurant, Daphne's. 'Good,' I said, 'I never go there.' Night weight 83kg.

FRIDAY 19 MAY

Morning weight 83.1kg or 13st 1lb. Note I've lost one kilogram overnight. It's all a near disaster! At 13 stone two pounds I will throw myself from the basement window. That is my absolute upper level. I should not have had the jelly at The Ivy last night – it's got sugar in it. Or the cream. Matters are made worse because today I fly to Lake Como. Italian food is the most difficult to avoid. Breakfast: goat's milk yoghurt, jam, clementine juice. Lunch sadly I forget but it wasn't much. Dinner at the Grand Hotel Villa Serbelloni in Bellagio on Lake Como. I am here with the lovely Geraldine. Very beautiful hotel and view. Small portions of steamed asparagus, cream, poached egg and truffle, wild duck cooked in two ways, plums filled with foie gras and spinach leaves. Tiny bit of white chocolate cake and capresi, a Naples cake made with chocolate and almonds. Night weight (on hotel scales, which I think flatter the situation) 83kg.

SATURDAY 20 MAY

Morning weight 81kg or 12st 10½lbs. I find this hard to believe. I think on my scales I'd be more but Geraldine has weighed herself and said it tallied with her scales in Milan, where she currently lives. (Remember, she's teaching dance there at her sister's dance studio. I much look forward to her returning to be with me when her term ends in July.) Breakfast: fresh orange juice, sliver of ham, small portion of bacon, scrambled eggs, cappuccino with no sugar, some mixed salami. (Geraldine said that was okay as long as I didn't have bread with it, which I didn't.) Lunch at Locanda dell'Isola Comacina, a restaurant on the only island in Lake Como. The wonderfully eccentric owner, Benvenuto Puricelli, wears a tartan waistcoat and hat. He did explain why but it was beyond me. When I first came here 10 years ago I had a blazing row with him and walked out. He pursued me and we became friends. I've since met him in Barbados. He was, naturally, overjoyed to see me and seated us outside overlooking a lovely little town. He produced a big, warm bread roll, very long. I only took a little from it. A big slice of tomato with lemon on the top and olive oil. A vegetable hors d'oeuvre of celery, cauliflower, courgette, tomato, carrots, beans and chicory. Then cuts from an enormous prosciutto of Praga. It's cooked and slightly smoked. Then dried beef bresaola. Big baked onion, fantastic taste! Still mineral water. Fresh trout grilled on a hotplate over charcoal. Free-range chicken fried in an iron pot with oil and served with salad. The same menu has been served here day and night since 1947! Then ice cream with banana liqueur and sliced oranges. Dinner at the Hotel Villa Serbelloni: prawns from San Remo, then mashed cod like a pâté, then a fish, lavarecco del lago, from Lake Como, then coffee ice cream made with liquid nitrogen. This caused endless hot ice smoke to billow everywhere, like at a rock concert or a pantomime. While we watched, Francesco the restaurant manager stirred the ice cream. As he poured in the liquid nitrogen more smoke billowed out. Then he crumbled a few cantucci biscuits on top and poured it into a large champagne glass over jelly. Geraldine said, 'Maybe liquid nitrogen is slimming.' I said, 'I doubt it!' Night weight 82.5kg.

SUNDAY 21 MAY

Morning weight 82kg or 12st 12¾lbs on the hotel scales, which I still think are more favourable to me than mine at home. Breakfast: scrambled egg, one piece of bacon, cappuccino, fresh orange juice, a piece of a croissant with jam and butter. Lunch at the Nilus Bar, Varenna on Lake Como. This was a 'drop in'. Varenna, is a beautiful, unspoiled village. The Nilus Bar is right on the water. We were on a boat trip around the lake. We'd even photographed George Clooney's villa. How touristy can you get? At the Nilus I had a very good pizza with tomato, mozzarella, rocket, sliced Parmesan. I was dictating details into my tape when a woman from Cheshire, with a rucksack, came over. 'Is this the BBC? Are you doing a book?' 'No, I'm just a poor tourist on holiday,' I advised. 'I won't see it on television then?' said the Cheshire lady. 'No,' I said. Then I had vanilla ice cream, which came on a plate the shape of a heart. And four tiny boiled sweets, which were at the cash desk. Geraldine said, 'You can't have sweets, you're diabetic.' I replied, 'I'm only border-line diabetic. Sweets are very good for borderline diabetics. They're well known for being good for them.' Dinner at the Villa Serbelloni. They recommended, and I accepted, an amuse-bouche of tartare of veal, then a vitello tonnato, which is a thin slice of veal with some tuna sauce. Then ravioli stuffed with ricotta cheese, herbs and one egg. It's gone bloody mad here! Then a third course of veal from Piemonte and underneath it artichokes and potatoes. I only ate about a third of it because I'm on a diet. Not that you'd notice! Followed by a chocolate pudding with vanilla sauce and small cherries. Night weight 83.5kg.

MONDAY 22 MAY
Morning weight 82.5kg or 13st. Breakfast: a yoghurt with jam, scrambled eggs, cappuccino. Lunch at Grand Hotel Villa Serbelloni: a club sandwich in four pieces. On skewers. I ate half of it. A vanilla ice cream. Cappuccino, no sugar. Dinner at Villa Serbelloni: asparagus, then scampi from Sicily with grilled vegetables. Dessert was a vanilla soufflé with vanilla sauce and chocolate sauce. This is not your normal diet food. Night weight 83kg. Amazing, I seem to have lost 0.5kg. Over a pound!

TUESDAY 23 MAY
Morning weight 82kg or 12st 12¾lbs. I have difficulty believing this, but it's definitely what the scales said! Breakfast at Villa Serbelloni: orange juice, cappuccino with no sugar, small amount of smoked salmon, cream cheese, cottage cheese and scrambled egg. Travelled to the old city of Bergamo on my way to Milan. Lunch in the 13th-century square of Bergamo at Trattoria Sant' Ambroeus: Bergamo ravioli with bacon and sage and then roast rabbit with roast potatoes instead of the advertised polenta. Then what they assured me was lemon ice cream, but tasted just like lemon sorbet.

Arrived at the very plush and well-run Four Seasons Hotel in Milan where, amazingly, there were no scales anywhere, in the bathroom or elsewhere. Dinner at Velo Bar, Via G da Procedo, Milan. This is a very simple place, plastic tables, a bar, ice cream on sale outside. It's a favourite of Geraldine's. I had too many potato crisps from a bowl on the bar. Meal was octopus salad, then a grain called faro with tomato and some sort of sauce, then penne with smoked cheese and meat, then the main course of small pieces of sea bass with thinly sliced fried zucchini (courgettes). Finally we had a toasted panettone topped with whipped mascarpone cheese, cream, eggs and sugar. Delicious. Perhaps luckily, could not check my night weight.

WEDNESDAY 24 MAY
No morning weight owing to no scales! On private jet from Milan: three small Mars sweets. Lunch at home: two goat's milk yoghurts totalling 250 grams, raspberries, brown granulated sugar. Party to celebrate 100 years of The Ritz hotel. I drank nothing. Ate one small canapé of pastry with some meat in it. Dinner at The Wolseley. Tiny bit of bread and butter. Still mineral water. 50 grams Beluga caviar – only had two very small blinis. Ate the rest with chopped egg, onion and sour cream off a knife until I found a sort of plastic spoon, then I used that. Steak tartare for main course with lettuce salad. Mint tea with real mint leaves and hot water, no sugar. Night weight (now on my scales at home) 84kg. Disaster but not unexpected.

THURSDAY 25 MAY

Morning weight 83.4kg or 13st 1¾lbs. Horrific! And I face dinner tonight out with friends. This is getting very dangerous indeed. Breakfast as usual: two goat's milk yoghurts of 125g each, some jam mushed in with them, fresh clementine juice. Lunch: two goat's milk yoghurts with raspberries. Dinner at Cecconi's with David and Wendy, who won't allow me to tell you their second name. He supplies supermarkets with things ranging from dried flower arrangements to perfumes bearing the names Elle McPherson and Normandy Keith. Wendy was in TV production and is now aiming for movies. They're about the only people in trade I bother to see. Cecconi's was owned by a man named Enzo Cecconi, who in my opinion is now a total bore. He lives in Venice and muscles in whenever he sees a celebrity. At my 70th birthday party he came up to Michael Caine, just intruded, and talked forever like he was Michael's best friend. When he left Michael said to me, 'Who was that?' When Enzo first opened Cecconi, he did a good job, but he let it slip down the toilet. It was bought by some people who ran it worse. It's now owned by a very nice and clever man, Nick Jones. He's pulled it up. I like it. Very buzzy. I ate some Italian sausage with peppers, a small portion of salmon tartare, then disaster – three scoops of vanilla ice cream. What a mindless idiot I am! I even had a tiny spoonful of a chocolate soufflé-type thing from the plate of one of my guests. Night weight 84.4kg. Even worse than yesterday! I am a total arsehole.

FRIDAY 26 MAY
Morning weight 83.5kg or 13st 2lbs. This is the worst! In fact, I'll tell you a secret. I'm cheating! My normal scales showed 83.6kg so I took the weight from the scales next to it! Am I slipping back to being a fat pig?! Is this the end of a beautiful moment in history? I must be firm and resolute. Breakfast: 450g yoghurt, more than usual, and a different kind – Rozbert organic live goat's milk bio yoghurt! With jam added by me. There's a Bank Holiday weekend coming. I'm due to go out a lot. This will be the test of whether I have willpower or not. I am shaking. 11-ish: coffee with Bailey's Irish Cream. Lunch (you won't believe this!): spaghetti bolognese with butter chucked on top and grated cheese. There's absolutely no question, I'm a f**king moron. I mean who, other than a moron, would eat spaghetti with butter when they're not only on a diet but creeping up to overweight again and writing a diet book? Do not do as I do. Show willpower. Although I'm planning a practically nothing-to-eat dinner, this is ridiculous. I'm hoping, when I weigh myself tomorrow morning, for a miracle loss of weight. I should be so lucky! We'll see! 4.30pm: coffee with a dash of 1977 (29-year-old) single malt Macallan Scotch whisky in it. I am drowning my sorrows at weight increase. Dinner: two raw carrots, two 125g Delamere live goat's milk yoghurts, raspberries, brown granulated sugar, still mineral water. Night weight 84.4kg.

SATURDAY 27 MAY
Morning weight 83.6kg or 13st 2¼lbs. So awful I am speechless. On 6 May, when I started this diary, I was 12

stone 12 pounds. So I've gained four and a quarter pounds in just over three weeks! Fear not, I'm determined to lose three pounds. Not cash, weight. Read on and you will see it happen! Breakfast: 225g Rozbert's organic live goat's milk bio yoghurt with jam, clementine juice. 11-ish: coffee with Bailey's Irish Cream and organic milk. Lunch at Scalini in Walton Street. Paul McKenna, the hypnotist and nice person, was there. I ate tomatoes in olive oil and herbs, grilled sole, fresh fruit salad, fresh mint tea. A few potato crisps at The Ritz hotel later. Dinner with Paola at The Ritz. They have a four-piece band. The grand Ritz dining room is something out of the 1930s. Candles reflect in vast mirrors, gilt chandeliers, painted sky on the ceiling. Very pleasant. I ate some little starter of scrambled egg in an eggshell with caviar, celery soup, lobster bisque, halibut in a creamy sauce. And then temptation took over and I had crêpes with Grand Marnier and two gooseberry cake petits fours with fresh mint tea. Ridiculous. Night weight a massive 85.3kg.

SUNDAY 28 MAY
Morning weight 84.3kg or 13st 3½lbs. I am one and a half pounds over my top weight limit! Disgraceful. I'm going out very little next week so I truly believe I can claw it back, thus demonstrating to you how all is possible. Today it broke in the newspapers that I'd turned down an OBE and said it was for people who clean toilets at railway stations. I didn't form The Police Memorial Trust to pay tribute to policemen slain on duty and I didn't put up a National Police Memorial in the Mall, which the Queen unveiled, to get an honour. I did

it because it seemed unfair the police were the only service fighting and dying – as do the Army, Navy and Air Force – who had no public recognition. Breakfast: 225g Rozbert's live organic goat's milk yoghurt with jam, clementine juice. Lunch at the Petersham Nurseries Café: tiny piece of bread and butter, still mineral water, their home-made lemonade. Orford's cod's roe with crème fraîche and sourdough toast. Chickpea, sweet potato and spinach curry with bhatura. Meringue with strawberries and cream. Fresh mint tea. Dinner at 8 Over 8, a ghastly restaurant in Chelsea with an utterly incompetent manager who first said they were full and I couldn't come and then relented. Once there I faced a large number of empty tables throughout the meal. And he didn't even know who I was, which didn't worry me at all! The service was slow to the point of ridiculous. The room is gloomy. Nothing whatsoever like the quality, charm, buzz and brightness of its sister restaurant, E&O in Notting Hill Gate. I ate lobster soup and a duck salad with peanuts and squash. In spite of this light dinner my night weight was a highly dispiriting 85.1kg.

MONDAY 29 MAY
Morning weight 84.3kg or 13st 3¾lbs. So even after my very modest dinner I still put on a quarter of a pound yesterday. The moral of this is, you have to be ever vigilant. No, super-vigilant. My aim is to be back at 13 stone or less by next Friday. Breakfast: goat's milk yoghurt, jam, clementine juice. Lunch today could have been a disaster because I had to go to The Wolseley. Derren Brown, Ed Victor, Rupert Everett and Lucian Freud

were there. In the 1950s I used to sit nearly every day next to Lucian and Francis Bacon at the bar of Wheeler's in Old Compton Street, Soho. So you could say we've known each other a long time. I ate a walnut and orange salad followed by 50 grams of Beluga caviar and then a peach sorbet. Dinner at 6.30pm: 250g of Woodlands live goat's milk yoghurt with raspberries and brown granulated sugar plus 125g Delamere live goat's milk yoghurt with jam. Night weight a suicide-inducing 85.5kg.

TUESDAY 30 MAY
Morning weight 84.7kg or 13st 4¾lbs. I don't understand this. Perhaps fruit and yoghurt at night, although I ate them at 6.30pm, are more fattening than I thought. Or perhaps it's the combination and accumulation of over-eating on the Bank Holiday weekend. I must pull back or we'll have to cancel the book and get 43 jackets let out when they've just been taken in! Plus trousers, plus... It's too awful to contemplate. I'm still well below the 15 stone ten pounds I used to be in the morning. But that's no consolation. Breakfast: 225g Rozbert organic live goat's milk bio yoghurt, plus jam I added. I wasn't going to add the jam but I weakened! My maximum weight should be 13 stone two pounds. I need to lose two and three-quarter pounds – quick! 11-ish (and this won't help!): coffee with Bailey's Irish Cream. Lunch: lamb cutlets, carrots, beans. It was rack of lamb. I ate far too much – and with mint jelly! I am a total idiot. In the afternoon the *Daily Mirror* brought round the most marvellous lady who is a toilet cleaner at King's Cross and her daughter, who works for the police. We had tea

in my house. They were both a delight. We got on marvellously. Hilma (the mother) can make curried goat, which was one of my all-time favourite meals in Jamaica. The day before the *Mirror* had, shall we say, encouraged her to say nasty things about me before she'd even met me. She obviously said nice things after leaving me because they didn't print the story of her visit to me at all. Instead one of their hack lady columnists just attacked me again for turning down the OBE and for saying it was for people who clean the toilets at King's Cross. I will write to the appointments secretary suggesting, quite seriously, that this lovely lady, named Hilma Daley, is given the OBE. She deserves it. She's an exemplary citizen. Dinner at E&O in Notting Hill: broth soup with noodles and cabbage, a few Chinese steamed vegetables. Still water. That was good. But I ate too much lamb at lunch. Night weight 85.6kg.

WEDNESDAY 31 MAY
Morning weight 84.9kg or 13st 5lbs. Very bad. Up a quarter of a pound. It's the lamb wot did it! My comfort zone is 12 stone 12 pounds to 13 stone two pounds. I ain't a million miles from it, but I ain't in it either. Today I will be very careful. The weight has to start going down tomorrow morning! Breakfast: 225g Rozbert organic live goat's milk yoghurt, jam, clementine juice. Lunch: cold crabmeat, a few lettuce leaves. PM: a small piece of Rococo sugar-free and dairy-free chocolate. Dinner: two raw carrots, two soft-boiled eggs. One chocolate biscuit. Night weight 84.7kg.

THURSDAY 1 JUNE

Morning weight 83.6kg or 13st 2¼lbs. A triumph! One day of seriously contained eating and I've lost two and three-quarter pounds! I must now keep it up – or down is perhaps a better word. Breakfast: Rozbert organic goat's milk yoghurt, jam, clementine juice. Lunch: grilled salmon, asparagus, hollandaise sauce. Dinner (this is odd!): started on private jet to Stockton-on-Tees, where I had to go to appear on the BBC's *Question Time*. On the way there I had a packet of Walker's crisps (plain of course) and three sandwiches – but these were like one sandwich cut into four and I had three pieces. They were quite bulky, though. Then in the Arc Centre, Stockton-on-Tees, I had three chocolate digestive biscuits and one cup of Earl Grey tea without sugar. On the drive to the airport for the return journey there were some toffees in the limo passenger door, so I had four of those. Then on the plane on the way back I had another packet of Walker's crisps and – at the last moment – an entire packet of Smarties! So I was surprised, and glad, to see my night weight was down from yesterday at 83.9kg.

FRIDAY 2 JUNE

Morning weight 83.2kg or 13st 1¼lbs. I've done it! I'm back in the comfort zone. Bit of a miracle, really. Or will I pay later for yesterday's Smarties, the crisps and the toffees? Breakfast: Rozbert organic goat's milk yoghurt, jam, clementine juice. 11-ish: coffee with Bailey's Irish Cream. Lunch: spaghetti bolognese with grated Parmesan and a big, and I do mean big, lump of butter chucked on top! Dinner at 6.30pm: two raw carrots, two lightly boiled eggs, three smallish chocolate biscuits. Night weight 83.5kg.

SATURDAY 3 JUNE

Morning weight 82.8kg or 13st ½lb. This is a triumph but I must tell you what happened at 2am, because it affects what I had for lunch. As I was lying in bed I scratched a tiny spot or scab on the front of my right leg, about six inches below the knee. Then I felt it bleeding. So I got up and held a handkerchief over it. It seemed to be bleeding profusely. I went to the bathroom off the bedroom. By the time I got there the handkerchief was totally sodden and dripping with blood. (The faint-hearted can skip this next bit!) I removed the handkerchief and blood poured out of my leg. I held face flannels against it. They were soaked in seconds. I stood up and saw what appeared to be a spider's web from my leg to the mirrored doors of my bathroom cabinets. I tried to 'whoosh' the spider's yarn away. The thin black line remained. Then I realised what it was. Blood was spurting from my leg in a thin stream like water from a tiny hole in a hosepipe. It splattered onto the marble floor two feet away! The whole floor was awash with blood. I thought, 'How do I deal with this? Will I bleed to death?' Every time I moved anywhere more blood poured onto the floor. Some years earlier I had a bedsore and I'd kept a lot of the para-phernalia associated with dressing it. I took about 20 layers of thin gauze from a bathroom drawer and put that on the tiny hole in my leg. It immediately seeped up blood. Then I took a bandage and wrapped it around and around. There I stood, with no way of fixing the bandage until I remembered I had some tape in a drawer outside the bathroom. I got it and wrapped it endlessly around the bandage. So now I had an enormous dressing around the wound. Blood did not seem to be coming through. Nervously I returned to bed, leaving the bathroom looking like six people had been slaughtered in the *Texas Chainsaw Massacre*. I would say well over a pint of blood lay in spatter patterns in the bathroom and on the cabinets. I tried to sleep but couldn't. I took half a Rohypnol. This is the so-called 'date rape' pill that is banned in England. I get it abroad. Now it's banned abroad too. I find it an excellent sleeping pill. This is what it is intended for. I slept. In the morning no more blood had come out. I spent an hour and a half on my knees cleaning the bathroom, wringing blood out of face flannels into the bath, the two sinks or the bidet, whichever was nearest. I called Depak Patel, the pharmacist at the Pestle and Mortar in Kensington High Street. He kindly came over with more bandages, more coverings and more reserve stuff in case it happened again. Even though weakened by loss of blood I had my usual breakfast: goat's milk yoghurt with jam and clementine juice. 9.30-ish: coffee with Bailey's Irish Cream. Then I went to sign my autobiography at an autograph fair in a hotel near Heathrow. Sir Norman Wisdom was the biggest attraction! I waited for his queue to get through and then many of them came on to me! There I had one coffee with milk and sugar. Then to The Wolseley in Piccadilly for lunch. I ate (feeling I needed building up!) one roll with butter, herring and cream cheese; lamb navarin, which is lamb and veggies and potatoes; and a fantastic piece of pie (which had a fancy name) to which I added whipped cream. Then a mint tea, no sugar. This is more than I would have eaten had I not needed to build up my reserves due to blood loss! Dinner: goat's milk yoghurt with raspberries and granulated brown sugar, plus three smallish chocolate biscuits. Night weight 83.6kg.

SUNDAY 4 JUNE
Morning weight 82.9kg or 13st ¾lb. Breakfast: goat's milk yoghurt with jam, mixture of orange and clementine juice. 11-ish: coffee with Bailey's Irish Cream. Lunch at Michael and Shakira Caine's. A dieter's disaster! Best food anywhere. Buffet of chicken, sausages, stuffing, boiled potatoes, mashed potatoes, mixed veg, gravy. For dessert cheesecake, various Häagen-Dazs ice creams, rhubarb picked by Michael in the garden that morning. I ate everything, preceded by a Pimms and some Doritos, and ending with mint tea with no sugar but three Turkish delight sweets and two chocolate mints. The President of Iceland was one of the guests. Oliver. Very nice person. I used to take out an Icelandic girl, very beautiful, way back in the 1950s. Oliver knew her and her mother and brother. Well, it's a small country, Iceland. He probably knows everybody. No dinner of any meaning tonight and it'll still be a disaster! Dinner at 6.30pm: goat's milk yoghurt, strawberries and granulated brown sugar. Night weight 84.5kg.

MONDAY 5 JUNE
Morning weight 83.8kg or 13st 2¾lbs. A two-pound increase because I pigged out at the Michael Caine lunch!

This illustrates caution is essential – faced with such marvellous food I threw caution to the winds. You mustn't do that. Eat all the stuff. Just eat less of it. Breakfast: goat's milk organic live yoghurt, jam, clementine juice.11-ish: coffee with Bailey's Irish Cream. Lunch: small grilled Dover sole, fresh peas, carrots, still mineral water. 4pm: coffee with Bailey's Irish Cream. Dinner: two raw carrots, two lightly boiled eggs. Note I had coffee with alcohol twice today! This is because I was under great stress caused by the cellular phone people at O_2. In 1984 I bought a British Telecom cellphone. It cost £3,300.00! Really, it did. Now I have six cellphones, three on Vodafone and three on O_2. It's useful to have both because you may be in an area where one of the companies hasn't got a nearby aerial but the other has! I keep one cellphone in each of my four cars and two loose in the office, which I take abroad with me. The six phones I had were very, very old – one was so used that the dial pad numbers were completely cracked and unidentifiable. Although they all still worked I decided to change the lot – Motorolas and Ericssons – for a simple Nokia. I didn't want a phone that takes photos, cooks dinner, sends emails to Mars – just a basic phone. My SIM cards were so old they fitted in the new phones – but didn't work! So I had to have six new SIM cards. The ones from Vodafone came with a little note explaining which phone number they related to. They were put online in five minutes. A very efficient operation. The ones from O_2 did not have a note saying which phone number they related to. Unlike Vodafone they were blocked. A sign came up saying 'Enter PIN number'. O_2 had not told me the pin number!

First time I rang they said '5555'. But that didn't unblock the phone. Second time I rang they said '8888'. That didn't unblock the phones either. The third time they said '4321'. You guessed it. That didn't work! After many more calls, getting increasingly fractious on my part, O_2 staff did manage to find their own unblocking code! It then took many more calls before anyone at O_2 could tell me how to take the need for a PIN block off the phone altogether. Five minutes to get the phones going from Vodafone. Four hours and endless calls to and fro with O_2. Yet I read Vodafone is vastly in debt! Arun Sarin, their chief executive, is my hero. I don't care what anyone else says! Anything remotely mechanical drives me into a frenzy anyway! I consider it an achievement if I can open the fridge. Dinner: two raw carrots, two soft-boiled eggs, three small chocolate biscuits. Night weight 83.4kg.

TUESDAY 6 JUNE
Morning weight 82.8kg or 13st ½lb. A triumph! One day of sensible eating, even though it included three chocolate biscuits and two coffees with Bailey's Irish Cream, and I've lost two and a quarter pounds! If I can do it, believe me, you can. Breakfast: Rozbert organic live goat's milk yoghurt with jam, clementine juice. Still aggravation with my new cellphones from O_2. The three Nokias from Vodafone rang when telephoned. Of the three from O_2, one rings, one shudders like a massage chair and one simply asks you to leave a message. Why on earth do O_2 send SIM cards out set like that? A nice man, Lee Kenley from Nokia, sorted it out. He had the marvellous title of Product Marketing Manager for

Independent Retailers and Distribution. He told me it wasn't the SIM cards, O_2 must have done it all by hand – that is making phones not ring! I hope that's over now. Back to my food intake. 11-ish: the inevitable coffee with Baileys Irish Cream. No, Bailey's do not give me the stuff so I can plug it. We buy it locally, not even discounted! Lunch: three small pieces of grilled plaice (I ignored the sauce tartare put out for it) and sweetcorn (I ignored the butter put out for it)! Also broccoli and still mineral water. One real chocolate filled with something or other. Great dinner: I took 100 grams of Beluga caviar and put it on a large plate. Lightly boiled three eggs, scooped the eggs out over the caviar and ate with knife and fork. Fantastic! I went mad and had a large glass of Vieux-Château-Certan Pomerol 1989 and then four smallish chocolate biscuits. The wine was chosen for me by Serena Sutcliffe, Master of Wine and head of the wine department at Sotheby's. She's a gem! I always say, 'Serena, I want three cases of wine from your next auction. You choose.' She buys three cases, twelve bottles in a case. They're always terrific. Wine at auction is about a quarter or less of the price you pay in a restaurant and about half the price you pay in a shop. And with Serena choosing it, which she may not do for you, it's always great. Night weight 83.4kg.

WEDNESDAY 7 JUNE
Morning weight 82.7kg or 13st ¼lb. A moderate triumph! Another day of getting weight down! Breakfast: goat's milk yoghurt, jam, clementine juice. 11-ish: coffee with Bailey's Irish Cream. My cook went on holiday this

morning. She's not back until 4 July. Normally when she's away I get a local chef, Billy Reid, from the nearby Belvedere restaurant in Holland Park, to come over and provide a one-course meal for my lunch. But he's so good I fear it will be too fattening. I was well down on all staff today – my chauffeur, who sometimes gets food for me, is also on holiday; Dinah May, my main, and outstanding, receptionist, only works two weeks on, two weeks off and she's off this and next week; and one of my other lady assistants is in Poland. Don't ask why. So Gae Exton, my remaining receptionist, went, as requested, and bought a salad from Marks & Spencer. It was fresh but it looked boring. So I foolishly added some Brie cheese, which is probably fattening, and some raisins. It was still extremely dull. I don't know what I'll do tomorrow. Oh yes I do. I have to go to lunch with the owner of Fortnum & Mason at their store. I just mustn't eat much. 4.30-ish: one ordinary chocolate – y'know, one of those single things from a box, in this case shaped like a top hat and from The Ritz hotel in Piccadilly. Dinner at 6.30pm: lovely 100 grams of caviar with three soft-boiled eggs scooped out and chucked on top. A little matzo, which is a sort of thin wafer biscuit, with butter, instead of my usual three chocolate biscuits. Then I had a smallish plate of raspberries. No sugar, no cream, just raspberries. Night weight 83.1kg.

THURSDAY 8 JUNE
Morning weight 82.4kg or 12st 13¾lbs. Yerss. Very good. Breakfast: the usual goat's milk yoghurt, jam, clementine juice. In February we had corresponded with Abel

Hadden, PR for Fortnum's, and I accepted an invite to lunch today. (They give Chairman's lunches from time to time. The Chairman is a lady called Jana Khayat.) So we rang them. The PR was away and the store said, there's no Chairman's lunch. It was obviously cancelled but nobody bothered to tell me! Typical of people in public relations. In the old days they said the idiot of the family went into the Church. Now the idiot of the family goes into public relations. Apparently they're completely re-designing Fortnum & Mason using a man whose designs are unbelievably tedious and ghastly, David Collins. They should realise it's a beautiful building inside and out. Other than the food, they're just selling the wrong stuff. Save a fortune on re-design, which is almost bound to leave it looking worse, and learn about retail, I say. And if you invite people to lunch, give the lunch! This left me without anything to eat. So Gae went to get a fruit salad from Marks & Spencer. It was very boring. It wasn't going off, or soggy, and it was sort of professional, but who cares? I think we sometimes get our organic vegetables from Marks. But they're cooked. Anyway, all I had was this M&S fruit salad. Then I desperately wanted something else. So I took a small, 50-gram bag of KP salted peanuts from the kitchen. (Paola had said we should get small containers of stuff because we were buying sizeable jars of jam and marmalade and nuts, and they'd get opened and then go off.) I know salted peanuts are fattening, but there weren't many of them. I was encouraged to read on the packet 'High in fibre. Source of vitamin B3. Naturally low in carbohydrate'. And then 'Nuts about nuts'. Oh well, we'll see the damage tomorrow morning, if indeed there is any. No diet can exclude everything we like or it'll never be pursued. At 4.20pm: one chocolate from The Ritz top hat! Dinner: 100 grams Beluga caviar, two soft-boiled eggs scraped out and mixed in with it, a tomato salad (prepared by me!) with olive oil, vinegar and lemon dressing topped with oregano, and raspberries without sugar or cream. Three small chocolate biscuits. Night weight 83.3kg.

FRIDAY 9 JUNE
Morning weight 82.4kg or 12st 13¾lbs. Bit disappointing that. I was hoping to lose at least another quarter of a pound. As it is, it's the same as yesterday. Still, it's well within my 'comfort zone' and I'm still over two and half stone less than I used to be! Breakfast: the usual goat's milk yoghurt, jam, clementine juice. I'd like to write a poem about that, but one doesn't easily come to mind. Usual coffee with Bailey's Irish Cream. Lunch was a total, unmitigated disaster. I sent the chauffeur to Harry Morgan's, a New York-type delicatessen in my least favourite part of London, St John's Wood. I asked him to get two bits of cold fried fish (cod), some pickled cucumber and some gefilte fish, which is a kind of cold fish ball. The fried fish for lunch, and the rest for dinner. He came back at ten to one and said, 'The fish is hot because they cooked it specially.' So I rushed downstairs and put it on a plate. But there weren't two bits of fish, there were four absolutely enormous pieces of fish. Superb. I decided to eat them all, piggy-Winnie returning. But I couldn't. So I put some in the fridge. Just as well because when I took out what I thought would be gefilte fish for dinner (at 6.30pm)

it wasn't as I remembered it. I thought gefilte fish was kind of white and soft. This was a fried fish ball. Undeterred I had two of them, plus some of the fried fish from lunch and some pickled cucumber. Nice meal. Had a second coffee with Bailey's in the afternoon as well! All this could do damage. 9.30-ish: one chocolate! Night weight 83.3kg.

SATURDAY 10 JUNE
Morning weight 82.7kg or 13st ¼lb. I only had fish yesterday, admittedly fried, and it put on half a pound. Not serious but it shows how careful you have to be. Good intentions are whittled away in tiny downward steps until you reach the bottom of the abyss. Tell you something else. After my breakfast of goat's milk yoghurt, bit of jam and clementine juice, I weighed myself again. I was 83.7kg. So just that little bit of liquid had put on three-quarters of a pound. Lunch at The Wolseley: hot white and green asparagus with hollandaise sauce, navarin of lamb with veggies and mashed potatoes, a peach sorbet. Took a walk in St James's Park in the afternoon. Watched *History of Violence* in my private cinema in the evening, a very good film. Followed by 250g of goat's milk yoghurt with jam (for a change) and, too late before bed, some cornflakes with Rachel's organic milk and brown sugar. I'll be disappointed if I don't stay at least the same weight. The late-arrival cornflakes were a mistake. Night weight 83.4kg.

SUNDAY 11 JUNE
Morning weight 82.5kg or 13st. A quarter of a pound down on yesterday. It's little triumphs like that which keep me

cheerful. Breakfast: goat's milk yoghurt, jam and clementine juice. 11-ish: coffee with Malibu, rum and coconut. No Bailey's, so I'd gone downstairs to the lounge drink's cupboard and found the Malibu there. It may well have been sitting around for 10 years or more. This tends to happen. I buy soft drinks, soda, that sort of stuff, never use them and they go past their sell-by date and get thrown out. I know liquor is supposed to keep but you should have seen my Warninck's advocaat after a 15-year sit. It was solid yellow muck. I threw a lot of bottles out of all sorts of stuff. Lunch at Scalini, which is a very, very good restaurant: tomatoes in oil and herbs, a little bread, few square bits of Parmesan, melon, wiener schnitzel (thin slices of veal in batter with capers, anchovies and a fried egg), fried zucchini, bit of salad, raspberries. Ate far too much. Felt bloated. Very bad. Dinner: one tomato sandwich, two small chocolate biscuits. Night weight 84.1kg.

MONDAY 12 JUNE

Morning weight 83.3kg or 13st 1½lbs. You see what damage one big meal can do! Up one and half pounds on yesterday morning! I'm a total moron. Breakfast: goat's milk yoghurt, jam, clementine juice. 11-ish: coffee with Bailey's Irish Cream. Lunch: 100 grams of Beluga caviar on two pieces of buttered brown toast, one small teaspoonful of smooth peanut butter, one small teaspoonful of crunchy peanut butter. Still mineral water. You think that's an odd lunch! Not for me it isn't! 4-ish: iced coffee with Bailey's Irish Cream. Dinner: fillet steak, tomato salad, two small chocolate biscuits. This'll be interesting. Have I lost a pound? Night weight 83.5kg.

TUESDAY 13 JUNE

Morning weight 82.9kg or 13st ¾lb. Well, I lost three-quarters of a pound. That's something. The scales this morning were madder than usual. When I got up at 5.50am (I'm a little early bird, aren't I?) I weighed 83kg. About 10 minutes later the same scales showed 82.9kg, three times. Then I did some gardening for 45 minutes. Ate nothing at all. When I came back and weighed myself I'd gone up to 83.2kg! An increase of 0.3kg, which is over half a pound – just through pottering about in the garden! Then five minutes later I weighed in at 83kg! Figure that out. I always take the lowest morning weight for these invaluable records. Breakfast: goat's milk yoghurt, jam, clementine juice. 11-ish: coffee with Bailey's Irish Cream. Piece of Rococo dairy-free, sugar-free chocolate. Lunch: 100 grams of Beluga caviar on two pieces of buttered brown toast. PM: a piece of Rococo chocolate. A glass of Vieux-Château-Certan Pomerol 1989 before dinner. I occasionally – not often – have a glass of wine in the evening. May not always have mentioned it before. Dinner: a disaster for my diet. At E&O in Notting Hill, a place I greatly like, I had chestnut and date gyozas, chicken and prawn dumplings, baby pork spare ribs, pad thai, which is (or was) noodles with soya, and chicken with some sort of crushed peanuts. A non-alcoholic fruit punch with mint, which I'm sure had a lot of sugar in it! Oh dear. But it's very jolly, E&O. Quite a buzz. Once when I saw Patsy Kensit there, she said she was fed up being a rock chick and could I find her a Jewish accountant. I said, 'Patsy, darling, that might be going a bit too far the other way.' My night weight was 83.2kg.

WEDNESDAY 14 JUNE

Morning weight 82.5kg or 13st. Breakfast: goat's milk yoghurt, jam, clementine juice. Lunch at the Soho Hotel for a pilot for a TV programme: tiny bit of focaccia bread, hot asparagus with hollandaise sauce, organic salmon with a half of one new potato, green beans, broccoli. A bit of appalling sticky toffee pudding, quite good small ice cream, a taste of raspberry trifle, fresh mint tea, one dreadful petit four. 4-ish: coffee with Bailey's Irish Cream. Dinner at Sticky Fingers. This was also for the TV pilot, a test for a series that may or may not happen. At Sticky Fingers, with ex-girlfriend Steffanie Pitt, I had samples only of potato skins with grilled cheese and some sauce, milkshakes of strawberry, vanilla, chocolate and banana, a chilli hamburger with chilli con carne on the side, a hot dog and a small sample of a chocolate brownie. Although it sounds grossly excessive I don't think I ate that much. Tomorrow's morning weight will tell the unavoidable truth. If I had to guess now I'd say I'll have put on half a pound. Night weight 83.4kg.

THURSDAY 15 JUNE

Morning weight 82.9kg or 13st ¾lb. So I put on three-quarters of a pound. Today will be a pull-back day. You have to have these now and then in order to keep weight down. And if you're trying to lose weight you need even more such days. You won't die from them. They become part of your life. They're the very minor price you have to pay for looking at a non-bloated, non-gross appearance when you see yourself in the mirror. Breakfast: goat's milk yoghurt, jam, clementine juice. 11-ish: coffee with

Bailey's Irish Cream. 12-ish: piece of Rococo sugar- and dairy-free chocolate. Lunch: 100 grams Beluga caviar on two pieces of buttered toast plus – wait for it! – two Actimel drinks in little plastic containers. Dinner: a grilled fillet steak, two water biscuits with butter and jam and an Actimel. Just before beddie-byes three tablespoonfuls of – guess what? – goat's milk yoghurt! Night weight 83.4kg.

FRIDAY 16 JUNE
Morning weight 82.6kg or 13st. Not bad. Breakfast: goat's milk yoghurt with jam (for a change!) and clementine juice. 11-ish: coffee with Bailey's Irish Cream. Have you got the impression I'm addicted to this? And to goat's milk yoghurt? Oh well, it's healthier than cocaine or heroin. Lunch: 100 grams of Beluga caviar on two slices of buttered toast, two Actimel drinks. Dinner at The Ivy. I had griddled foie gras, a Buck's Fizz and rhubarb crumble. The boss of The Ivy, Mitchell Everard, had left a few weeks ago, as did one of the senior managers, and they've got a new man there from Zuma as overall manager-boss of the group. He's very elegant, very charming. I couldn't fault him. He carried plates, he chipped in, he was welcoming. He's tall and good-looking. But there's a slightly different aura about the place. More staff will be dispersed when the comparatively new owner, Richard Caring, opens Scott's in Mayfair. I remember The Ivy when it was an 'in' place in the 1950s and 60s. Then it went down the tubes. After Chris Corbin and Jeremy King acquired it, they brought it back. I think restaurants have to be very careful not to spread themselves too thin. The Ivy is, rightly, the most

massively booked and popular restaurant in London. I greatly like it. I'd be sorry if it were to slide again. Night weight 83.2kg.

SATURDAY 17 JUNE
Morning weight 82.3kg or 12st 13½lbs. Breakfast: goat's milk yoghurt, jam, clementine juice. 10-ish: coffee with Bailey's Irish Cream. Helicoptered down to Andrew Lloyd Webber's Sydmonton estate for his TV show about finding a girl to play the lead, Maria, in his production of *The Sound of Music.* Andrew has lost two stone and he looks very skinny. He said he did it by swimming every evening in his indoor pool before going to bed. I think he must have cut down massively on food and drink as well. I'm told he lost the weight because he was to be seen on TV for weeks on end and didn't want to look fat and bloated. Whatever starts you on the road to slimness and sanity doesn't matter. Just start! Andrew had arranged for 10 girls to be on the stage in his church, adapted to a theatre. This was followed by lunch, which was catered by Mustard, who are irresistibly good. I was first at the buffet – nothing unusual about that! I took roast beef, one new potato, asparagus and a small fishcake. I'd eaten a few cheese straws before the audition started. My dessert was a small treacle tart, a small sorbet and some sweet biscuits. Plus black coffee, no sugar. Then we saw 10 more girls 'auditioning' for the role. They were all very good. Then tea. I had three egg finger sandwiches and a medium piece of carrot cake with cream. All too much. But over by 4.30pm. Dinner at 6.30pm: I held back. I only had – you've guessed it – goat's milk yoghurt

and jam. Then, encouraged by Geraldine, I walked for three-quarters of an hour in Holland Park. Night weight 83kg.

SUNDAY 18 JUNE
Morning weight 81.9kg or 12st 12½lbs. I think this loss of one and a quarter pounds following a day when I ate rather a lot is because I ate nothing after tea at 4.30pm other than my usual goat's milk yoghurt. I'm very pleased with this. When you become a serious dieter like me and your wife is amazed at how good you look (or if you're a woman then your husband is amazed at how good you look) these little achievements, day by day, are a source of real pleasure! Because I am not, thus far, slipping back into fattiedom. Breakfast: goat's milk yoghurt, jam, orange juice. Major departure here! Not clementine juice, orange juice. 'Why?' you ask. Because it's Sunday and my housekeeper's off, so I do the juice with my very own hand. Also, the oranges are larger so it's easier as I don't have to squeeze so many to produce the same amount of liquid! When you drink orange juice that was squeezed a few minutes before you drink it, you realise, in spades, how awful the so-called fresh orange juice is that is served in most restaurants. This in fact comes in a plastic carton and is stored in the fridge. It also tastes unbelievably better than juice squeezed on the premises in the restaurant and then stored before serving to the customer. Orange juice deteriorates within a very short time of being squeezed. At one of my favourite restaurants, Scalini in Knightsbridge, I always enjoyed their lunchtime orange juice. Then I was in one evening

and at 7.45pm they served me orange juice. It tasted nothing like the stuff they gave me at lunch. On investigation (I'm very good at restaurant investigations!) I discovered they squeezed their juice at 12.30pm. So my 7.30pm orange juice had stood around for seven hours deteriorating. I now ask very specifically in restaurants (a) if they've got real oranges and can squeeze them by hand (to illustrate that I make a squeezing motion with my hands) and (b) can they squeeze it now, as I wait. Sometimes it's a 'yes'. Sometimes a 'no'. If it's a 'no' I don't have it. Lunch today at Queen's Club for the finals of the Stella Artois Tennis Championships, at a 'do' given by Sir Frank Lowe, an advertising guru and exceptionally nice person. Sir Cliff Richard was there. I know it's a cruel thing to say, but it looks to me like he's had a lot of plastic surgery, which gives him the appearance of someone from outer space. I've always resisted plastic surgery. I can think of few people, if any, it makes look better. Food and beverage started with a Pimms and two sausages on sticks as canapés, then a buffet from which I took salmon, mayonnaise (the sort of pink-stuff mayonnaise), prawns and shrimps, no veg. Dessert was strawberries, raspberries and clotted cream. Then to the tennis, where an American called Blake was firmly and speedily beaten by Leyton Hewitt of Australia. Not much of a game really and over very quickly. So I could go back to the reception area for tea. There I ate two brown bread egg finger sandwiches, a small iced sponge cake, one mouthful of scone, jam and cream, three pieces of fudge, and a cup of tea, no sugar. This last food finished by 4pm. No dinner, for sure, except goat's milk yoghurt and jam. Evening weight 82.4kg.

MONDAY 19 JUNE

Morning weight 81.8kg or 12st 12¼lbs. Interesting that. Yesterday and the day before I ate quite piggishly at lunch and tea. Yet both days I lost weight. This is because after 4.30pm on Saturday and 4pm on Sunday I had nothing but goat's milk yoghurt and jam. And that was taken at 6.30pm. It shows how important it is to eat very little in the evening and also to eat it early. Look, there's no gain without pain. But I feel no pain at all. And I'm over two and a half stone thinner. Are you? No. Then shut up and get on with it. Breakfast: goat's milk yoghurt, jam, clementine juice. 11-ish: usual coffee with Bailey's. Lunch: two pieces of buttered toast with Beluga caviar, two little Actimel drinks. 4-ish: coffee with Bailey's. Before dinner I had a bit of Rococo dairy-free and sugar-free chocolate. This is rather good. It certainly tastes like chocolate. Dinner at 6.30pm. I'm boxing clever. Thought I'd have a change. Geraldine said to me over the weekend, 'You need more green vegetables.' Not mad about them. Anyway I made a dip (her recipe) of Philadelphia cream cheese, lot of olive oil, salt, oregano and other herbs, and lemon juice. I mushed it all up like a very junior league Gordon Ramsay. Then – wait for it! – I dipped into this substance one organic raw carrot. I ate all of that and then some raw broccoli. I ate the entire 'doctored' package of Philadelphia cream cheese, some of it with a fork. Then I had four small chocolate biscuits. Night weight 82.1kg.

TUESDAY 20 JUNE

Morning weight 81.6kg or 12st 11¾lbs. Still losing! Breakfast: goat's milk yoghurt, jam, clementine juice. Today I'm going to a Jewish funeral. In Golders Green, no less! It's for the lovely mum of Robert Earl, he who started and still owns Planet Hollywood and many other restaurants. They've got a lunch reception in a deli-catessen. This is not good for the diet. Maybe I should order an extra coffin for me. Perhaps if I order early I could do a deal. Get a discount. I'm a great believer in the Woody Allen philosophy, as expressed in a film he did with Diane Keaton. They're eating and she says, 'In my family it's considered bad manners to put your elbows on the table.' Woody replies, 'In my family it's considered bad manners to buy retail.' I was the first to leave the funeral service and area. Lunch was being served at Madison's Deli in Temple Fortune, or to be more precise in Finchley Road. I was the first there. The large room was laid out with a lot of food on the tables. There was sitting space for all. I sat down. I waited. But no one else turned up. I thought, 'I'll eat.' So I had a bit of chopped liver on rye bread, a falafel or two, some humus on the same rye bread and some pickled cucumber. After about 15 minutes other people from the funeral service came, including Robert Earl. Sir Philip Green sat opposite me. Robert assured me what was on the table was only the first course. I'd eaten enough to feel satisfied and leave. But this was not to be. Some frankfurter sausages arrived. I had one. Some latkes (potato pancakes) arrived. I sampled a little bit. Some salt beef arrived. I sampled a bit. Then Robert Earl said, 'You must try the lokshen pudding.' This is a very heavy Jewish pudding. It's so heavy people say 'You're making a lokshen pudding of this,' meaning someone is making heavy weather of something. So I waited until a hot lokshen pudding arrived, mercifully without the vanilla ice cream I'd been told was coming with it. I only had a tiny bit and it wasn't that heavy. Then I went home. Worried about my weight! Dinner at E&O in Notting Hill: walnut and date gyozas (two), prawn and chive dumplings (two), tiny bit of clear soup with mushrooms, black cod, Chinese veggies, a coconut sorbet. I love E&O. Night weight 82.3kg.

WEDNESDAY 21 JUNE

Morning weight 81.7kg or 12st 12lbs. A gain of quarter of a pound. Not bad! But I always wonder if you eat too much (as I did yesterday), does it hang over for the next 48 hours and come out to frighten you the day after the day after, if you get my drift. Breakast: goat's milk yoghurt, jam, clementine juice. 11-ish: coffee with Bailey's. Pre-lunch: small piece of Rococo dairy- and sugar-free chocolate. Lunch: two pieces of buttered toast with Beluga caviar. After lunch I had to go to do the Terry Wogan TV show. I put on a Brioni blazer that was marked 'Taken in in 2005'. It was much too big. I turned to a Doug Heywood (very 'in' tailor) blazer, also taken in by my alterations tailor in 2005. That was too big! So I had to wear a blazer made in June 1988 by my old tailor Maxwell Vine. It was one I'd rescued from the attic, where it had hung for years, never expecting to be worn again. The other two will have to be taken in for a second or third time. I thought, 'But if I take everything in to my current weight, what if I put on half a stone?' Think not like that! I am determined not to put on weight. I will not provide for a fat Winner! Terry Wogan, who is definitely overweight, bless him, said, 'Do you keep the weight off?' I said 'Yes. My book will tell you how to do that.' Terry said, 'I'll buy a copy.' 'I'll send you one,' I said. 'No,' said Terry, 'I'll buy one.' Hope he does! If it works for him it will be a thoroughly good investment of a few pounds (sterling). Dinner at 7pm. This may not be clever! One packet of Philadelphia cream cheese with added olive oil, a sliced banana, lemon juice, raspberries and brown sugar. All sort of mushed in a bowl! One chocolate biscuit. Night weight 82.1kg.

THURSDAY 22 JUNE

Morning weight 81.3kg or 12st 11¾lbs. This is the lowest I've been for years and years. Lost three-quarters of a pound since yesterday morning. Goodness, I'm clever! I was a bit worried the banana last night might have been a mistake. Some people say fruit at night is bad because there's sugar in it. But then people will tell you all different things about dieting. The proof is, what does what you eat do for you. Keeping a 'once a fat pig diary' like this tells all, incontrovertibly. 11-ish: coffee with Bailey's. Lunch: two pieces of buttered toast spread with Beluga caviar and one chocolate biscuit. 5pm-ish: bit of Rococo dairy-free and sugar-free chocolate. My alterations tailor came to take in jackets, some for the third time. He took away 12 jackets for this procedure. May this joy be yours. It will if you heed this book. It won't if you stay fat and ridiculous. Dinner: Philadelphia cream cheese mixed with olive oil, oregano, lemon juice and pepper. Into this I cut three organic tomatoes in little pieces. At the same time I munched an organic raw carrot. This may sound dreadful, but I found it very enjoyable! Then I had a big treat. (Not another chocolate biscuit.) At the lunch after the funeral I attended on Tuesday I had been recommended lamb's milk yoghurt by Anita Land. She's Jeremy Paxman's agent and daughter of one of the great agents of all time, Leslie Grade, brother to Lew Grade and Bernie Delfont. This lamb's milk organic yoghurt was very good. I plonked a spoonful of marmalade in and whooshed it about. The lamb's milk yoghurt is a bit creamier than goat's milk and I think it's a smoother taste. I'm leaning towards it. The nation waits breathlessly to see if I switch from goat's to lamb's. Little lamblets on the hills are saying to each other, 'Will we be the ones to provide milk for Michael Winner?' They'll have to wait, too. Night weight 81.7kg.

FRIDAY 23 JUNE

Morning weight 80.9kg or 12st 10¼lbs. You think this is easy, don't you? You think I just get on the scales in the morning and tell you my weight. Oh yeah! Take this morning. I got up at 6am. Weighed myself. Weight 79.7kg. I weighed myself again at 6.30am. I'd eaten nothing, drunk nothing. My best scales, which have the ridiculous name of BaByliss, now reported I was 81.2kg! Then I did a bit of early morning gardening, still without eating or drinking anything, and at 7.41am the scales said I was 80.9kg. Five minutes later, according to BaByliss, I weighed 81.1kg! At 8.11am I was 81kg. Still no food or drink had passed into my gorgeous frame. At 8.20am I was 80.9kg! Normally I would have taken the first weight which it showed twice after I got on the scales and off again. But as that was 79.9kg and all the others wobbled about, and as 80.9kg appeared twice on the morning weigh-in fiasco, that's the one I've chosen to report. After eating my breakfast of goat's milk yoghurt with marmalade chucked in it, and clementine juice, my weight had risen at 8.40am to 81.5kg. By 8.53am it had gone down to 81.3kg! This could drive anyone totally nuts! So I did my Pilates exercises, only to be interrupted around 9.05am by LBC's Nick Ferrari talk show. They wanted me to comment on some report that men were getting to be more like women. I was asked to say they weren't. The excellent writer and bright person Kathy Lette was on the show, all done on the phone. I was able to say, with great truth, that I was less like a woman than I had been because usually I had the biggest breasts on the beach in Barbados. Thanks to my two and a half stone (more today, actually!) weight loss, my breasts had now shrunk. Not gone completely, but shrunk. As indeed have I. And if you use a little willpower and take note of this book, so will you. 11-ish: coffee with Bailey's Irish Cream. Lunch: 220g of Plas Farm organic cottage cheese with a small Wilkin & Sons jar of blackcurrant jam whooshed in it and one sliced banana in there too. One chocolate biscuit. Now I bet you're saying, 'Just a minute! Winner said this diet was easy. Eat what you like. He's pouring in goat's milk yoghurt, sheep's milk yoghurt and now organic cottage cheese. This is not my idea of a fun lunch!' Strangely enough I would have said the same if I was reading another diet book. But we're approaching the weekend, when I'll be eating out again. Then next week I'm going to Portofino, where the food is historic. My old doctor used to say, 'Sleep is like money in the bank.' I say to you: on days where it's not 'essential' to eat fattening stuff, don't eat it. Lose a few extra pounds, so when you're tempted, as I will be in Portofino, you'll have a few pounds you can afford to put on. Funnily enough, and this does kind of amaze me, I don't feel denuded of more substantial food. I'm not hungry. I feel I've eaten enough. I do admit last night after my very early dinner of Philadelphia cream cheese, tomatoes, a raw carrot and lamb's milk yoghurt, I was a bit peckish around bedtime. But I simply had a glass of Malvern still mineral water and went to bed. In the old days I'd have sneaked down to the kitchen and knocked off at least one tub of vanilla ice cream! But then I was a fat pig. Now I look adorable. At least that's my delusion. About 5pm: small piece of Rococo chocolate. Dinner: lamb's milk yoghurt (I've decided it's definitely a nicer taste than goat's milk – I shall switch) with jam and then a fillet steak with two grilled tomatoes. And a few water biscuits with butter. Then I went to dinner (officially, but I only drank water) at the Hilton Hotel, Park Lane. The National Police Memorial, which I erected in the Mall, was being given an award from the Royal Institute of British Architects. It was, very strangely, put in the Arts and Leisure category. How 3,000 dead policemen count as 'Arts and Leisure' I can't imagine. Not only that, I didn't get the award! Spencer de Grey of Foster and

Partners (Lord Foster designed the memorial for my charity, The Police Memorial Trust) explained that they only announce the awards at the Hilton. He and I stood silent as the citation was read out. Then we shook hands with the President of the RIBA and had our photo taken with him. The award is actually to be presented in November! This is because the architects want it done region by region – I assume so they can be heroes in their own local press. About 10.30pm: small piece of Rococo chocolate. Night weight 81.6kg.

SATURDAY 24 JUNE
Morning weight 80.7kg or 12st 10lbs. Breakfast: goat's milk yoghurt, jam, clementine juice. Although I've decided to switch from goat's milk yoghurt to lamb's milk yoghurt, there are quite a few cartons of goat stuff (which I don't dislike) that I have to get through first. When I started my eating diary nearly seven weeks ago, on 6 May, I weighed 12 stone 12 pounds. It held more or less and then ballooned to a maximum of 13 stone five pounds on 31 May. But devouring the food intake I have listed for you, it speedily dropped to today's highly respectable low of 12 stone 10 pounds. So it shows, beyond doubt, this diet works! I am not putting weight back on. And when I do I go into action and get it off – fast! Believe me, you can do this. You can. You can. You can. Your wife will stop looking at you as an undesirable slob. Your children will show greater respect. If you're a woman you'll look in the mirror and see how useless all those beauty products are compared to losing weight. Your husband will desire you again. For now, keep

reading and see if I can maintain a slimline (all right, slimmish) Michael. 11-ish: coffee with Bailey's. Lunch at The Wolseley: very good but I pigged out. Started with a whole white bread roll with butter. Then a non-alcoholic fruit drink. Then herring with crème fraîche. I ate a bit of Paola's stuff, sort of crispbread something or other. Main course, boiled halibut and spinach. At this point Matt Lucas from the TV show *Little Britain* came to sit at the table next to me. I was with him on Reeves and Mortimer's *Shooting Stars,* when he banged the drums and announced the scores. Later I put some money in a West End musical by Boy George that Matt starred in. He was absolutely brilliant but I lost my money anyway. For dessert I had summer pudding (large portion) and cream. That was piggish. Went for a walk in Holland Park in the afternoon. Can't say it was vastly energetic but it was movement. Dinner: lamb's milk yoghurt with jam and some boiled broccoli with olive oil and vinegar. Watched a movie in my home cinema called *Me and You and Everyone We Know.* It wasn't terrible, but it was one of those movies that took itself far too seriously. And went on forever. You felt like screaming, 'Okay, we get the point, get on to the next scene!' Then I noted it won the Special Jury Prize at the Sundance Film Festival and three prizes at Cannes. It was the sort of film that said, 'I'm a festival entry, gimme something.' Bloody amazing they did! Around 9.45pm: strawberries with lemon juice. And occasionally during the day very small pieces of Rococo chocolate! Night weight 81.7kg.

SUNDAY 25 JUNE

Morning weight 81kg or 12st 10½lbs. See, I've put on half a pound. That's what happens when you have a white bread roll with butter and a large portion of summer pudding with clotted cream for lunch. Breakfast: goat's milk yoghurt and jam, orange juice (note orange, not clementine). 11-ish: coffee with single malt Strathmill Scotch whisky distilled in April 1963 and a small amount of brown crystal sugar. Great significance in the switch to whisky. I've run out of Bailey's Irish Cream. Must arrange to get it wholesale. Lunch at Scalini. Very good. Some little square bits of Parmesan cheese, some raw tomato with olive oil, a piece of bread, no butter, melon, a grilled sole, salad with oil and vinegar dressing, a few fried courgettes, a lemon sorbet. Scalini is one of my favourite places but it's dreadfully noisy. My corner table is in a good position but it's sandwiched between two large round tables. They can have as many as six people on each. Possibly eight. So not only are you close to the next group, very close, also their noise is upon you. So I said to the excellent restaurant manager, Michel Lengui, 'What is the number of that table?' I pointed to another table, theoretically not in as good a place as my usual table, but not hemmed in by groups. Michel gave me the number. All restaurant tables have a number known by the staff. I then said to the senior restaurant manager, Valerio Calzolari, 'It's so noisy here, I may want to try that table.' Valerio couldn't hear me. 'What did you say?' 'Exactly Valerio,' I said, now talking louder. 'I may want to try out table number...' and I gave the number. (Not telling you, you'll all want it.) He said, 'You won't like that table as much. The waiters walk by with the food.' 'Yes,' I said, 'I can see that. But at least there's space around it.' 3.30pm: I ate a piece of brown bread with butter and jam. This is because I forgot to take the 23 pills I normally take with lunch and needed a bit of food to go with them. Dinner: cottage cheese with jam and organic rapsberries. Then – very naughty this – a small pack of salted peanuts. I guess I'll put on another half a pound, which is definitely not clever. We'll see tomorrow. Night weight 81.8kg.

MONDAY 26 JUNE

Morning weight 81kg or 12st 10½lbs. A miracle. It's the same as yesterday in spite of a bit of binge eating! Breakfast: goat's milk yoghurt, jam, clementine juice. 10.30: coffee with Macallan single malt Scotch whisky distilled May 1977. (Note this is a different single malt to the whisky I used with my coffee yesterday, although it's not a vital point in regards to my diet!) 12.50pm: a single chocolate from the little top hat of chocolates from The Ritz hotel that sits on a ledge by my desk. Lunch: a cocktail, handmixed by me, of goat's milk yoghurt and sheep's milk yoghurt in the very same bowl! To that I added marmalade and a sliced banana. Who says dieting isn't exciting! Then I looked around for something else to eat, my cook still being away in the Philippines. I settled for a small packet of KP dry-roasted peanuts. This pack was brown. The blue pack I ate last night was labelled 'Original Salted Peanuts'. Does this mean these roasted ones aren't salted? They certainly tasted salted. If they are salted, why do KP keep it a secret? If they're not, why do I think they are? Any help you can give, please do. To digress... Have you noticed how little I go out? You have had a daily account of my eating for the last 52 days, including today, when I am out in the evening. So, counting today, I've eaten out of my house for only 27 meals in the UK out of a total of 94 UK meals. Well over two-thirds of my lunches and dinners are eaten at home! I'm not counting my trip to Lake Como in this highly significant calculation, because if you go abroad you're out all the time, aren't you? I am close to a recluse. A sort of touring version of Howard Hughes (a tiny bit saner). Roaming around my vast mansion alone. Sad it isn't. I'm very happy with my own company. People say to me, 'You must be out all the time!' To review a restaurant every week you only need to eat out an average of once a week. Even stay-at-homes do that. The press often refer to me as a 'boulevardier'. Anything less boulevardier than me I can't imagine. If I was, I'd give boulevardiers a bad name. I turn down endless dinner parties and events. Why should I commit myself to entertain people I don't know and who I may not like? Why should I stand with a mass of men and women holding drinks and looking for canapés? People say, 'Come to dinner.' I ask, 'Who else is coming? Who am I sitting next to?' 'My best friends are coming,' was one reply. What does that mean to me? Nothing! Then I was told who the best friends were. 'I'd rather watch the spin dryer,' I said. I guess I'm just a homebody. Having said all that, I was out at Le Caprice tonight for a disastrous (because I ate so much) dinner. Beforehand I had a glass of red wine (Cos-d'Estournel Saint Estèphe 1995) at home with my assistant Dinah. At

Le Caprice I had a bread roll with butter, a Buck's Fizz, asparagus with hollandaise sauce, a fishcake with spinach and extra sauce and, if that wasn't enough – which it was – I had some sort of gooey mousse with a chocolate ice cream sitting next to it! And grabbed bits of cheese and biscuit from Dinah. What a moron! I'm trying to keep my weight down. I bet this puts on two pounds tomorrow morning. This is just what you should not do. At least cut out the bread and the dessert. Or have a tiny bit of someone else's. If I'd done that I'd still have had a substantial meal. As it is I feel stuffed and stupid. At the same time! By the way, Salman Rushdie was there with his tall and beautiful young wife (they have since announced they are divorcing). It's rather like seeing Gandhi at a custard pie contest. As for Le Caprice, I remember it well in the 1950s, when I first came out on my own as it were. Then, if there was a theatrical first night, everyone wore evening dress. Le Caprice, under owner Mario Gallati, who named it after his wife's brassière, was the place to be. It had red plush seats and you entered from Arlington House, the block of flats it is attached to. The best seating area was where the door and bar are now. There was an alcove where are now the kitchens, sort of out of the way. Jews were placed there. That's true! I avoided the Caprice ghetto as I was a walker for an ageing lady theatrical agent. I worked as an agent briefly when I came down from Cambridge University. My salary was £10 a week. My secretary got £12.50. Monti Mackey, the ageing lady, bless her, worked in the same office. She was highly important. We represented James Mason, Richard Attenborough, Jack

Hawkins, Diana Dors. Monti took me to first nights and other events. (We didn't have a 'do' together! It was platonic!) At Le Caprice you'd have Laurence Olivier and Vivien Leigh on one side, over there would be Noël Coward, at that table Ivor Novello, there was David Niven and there Rex Harrison and Kay Kendall. All in evening dress. All very elegant. It was another world where a first-class meal at the 'in' place, Charco's in Chelsea, with steak and wine, cost 15 shillings all-in for two people. That's 75p in today's money. There were no parking problems, no yellow lines. You could drive up to the Empire cinema in Leicester Square, park your car by the box office, get out and go in. So few people had cars that defined parking spaces were not needed. Ah, but I'm dreaming. Le Caprice, re-born with its David Bailey celebrity photos and everyone looking like scruffs compared to the 1950s – none scruffier than me – is still a pleasure to visit. Except now I have to – or should – watch what I eat. In those days I could eat anything and never put on weight. After that heavy Caprice nosh my night weight was 82kg.

TUESDAY 27 JUNE
Morning weight 81.1kg or 12st 10¾lbs. I'm surprised! That's only half a pound up from yesterday after my highly incautious dinner last night at Le Caprice. I guess scales don't lie. I'm doing an article for the *Daily Mail* that involves me buying food that a pensioner, on £8.49 a day for everything except council tax, water and electricity bills, would eat. So I went to my local Waitrose with my assistant Dinah. We spent £11.62 on food,

which means £5.81 a day, leaving the remaining £2.68 a day for the pensioner to buy everything else with. From that food I made breakfast: one slice of Waitrose medium white sliced bread with Waitrose sunflower spread and Waitrose thin-cut Seville orange marmalade, plus two Stonegate straw-bedded eggs ('Hens bedded on straw with ample space to scratch, preen and dust bathe. Eggs of different sizes'). For breakfast I boiled those. They certainly were of different sizes. One vanished into my egg cup, hardly enough above egg-cup level to permit me to take the shell off. The next one stood proud! They both seemed to have more white and less yolk than the organic eggs I'm used to. But then we'd bought the cheapest possible of everything. Also Waitrose medium-roast instant coffee with semi-skimmed milk. I cheated and added some of my own crystal brown sugar. Then, after I'd eaten and drunk all of it, to take the mediocre taste away I cheated again and squeezed three of my own oranges! 11am: my lovely Blue Mountain coffee, from freshly ground beans, with 1977 single malt Macallan Scotch whisky. What a difference from the Waitrose medium-roasted instant. Mine smells fantastic, theirs smells like chemicals. Mine tastes marvellous, theirs dreadful. Thank God I can afford the best. I am ever grateful for that and, above all, good health! I then had two lunches! Not the best thing to do for a man on a diet! The first one was at home, where I ate the 'pensioner' food Dinah and I bought in Waitrose. I had salmon steak, broccoli, one grilled tomato, one jacket potato, sunflower spread and strawberries. I didn't eat all of anything, just enough to taste, although there wasn't much taste in any of it. Except the cheap, half-price, not organic Waitrose strawberries tasted much better than my organic ones, also from Waitrose, which cost much more. Then I had to have a second lunch with my friend Matthew Norman. He used to write the *Guardian Diary*, now he's the *Guardian* food critic, and does other columns everywhere. He's very funny and irreverent. We went to Assaggi, a small restaurant above a pub in Notting Hill. I inadvertently discovered this place 10 years ago. Dinah, my assistant, had it recommended to her by her ex-husband's brother. I expected nothing. But it was brilliant. I raved about it. Other food writers went and raved about it. Assaggi became very significant and now has a Michelin star. Nino, the co-owner and chef, was on duty. He just did a salad for me. Then I spoiled it by having some sort of poached peach with ice cream. And fresh mint-leaf tea. Matthew is a great fan, as I am, of Bernard Manning. Matthew used to go to his shows quite a lot. I joined with Robert Earl to pay for Bernard Manning to come down and do a cabaret at Marco Pierre White's 40th birthday party in a private reception room at his Mirabelle restaurant. I introduced Bernard effusively, describing him as one of the great comics of his generation. Bernard entered to applause. His first words were: 'Michael Winner, the most hated Jew in Europe.' I thought that was hilarious. Matthew reminded me of another Manning joke, which we both liked but you may not. Bernard said, 'I'm not racist. I believe we should all get together. The Blacks, the Chinese, the British, the Jews, the Italians, the French, we should all get together – and kick the shit out of the Pakistanis.' Dinner was on my pensioner £5.81 per day food stint. I had loin of pork, which was exceptionally good and very cheap (£1.90), a grilled tomato, some broccoli and strawberries. After dinner Jeremy King, co-owner of The Wolseley, rang me. Some Russian woman had booked a table for 4 July, saying I was going to be with her and the table was for me. Was it true? It wasn't. I always book restaurant tables myself in my own voice. Again and again people use my name to get into restaurants. I get irate letters from restaurateurs as far away as Devon and Scotland saying, 'Dear Mr Winner, you reserved for a party of eight last Thursday and you never showed up. Are you aware of what appalling manners that is …' Yes, I am. But if people use my name I can't help it. At one time some idiot was going around ordering Rolls Royce motor cars in my name. Jack Barclay and other famous show-rooms would ring up and say, 'Mr Winner, your Rolls is ready now. When would you like to collect it?' They were somewhat disappointed when I said I had two already and I honestly didn't order a third. Night weight 82.1kg.

WEDNESDAY 28 JUNE

Morning weight 81.5kg or 12st 11½lbs. An increase of three-quarters of a pound. Not good, not horrific. Break-fast: 200g sheep's milk yoghurt, jam, clementine juice. I'm off to Portofino today and some of the best food in the world. This will be a real test! Still, Geraldine is joining me there. She's bound to force me to walk an hour every evening. Around Portofino it's all up steep hills and down steep hills. It should help. Problem with my flight out! I was due to leave RAF Northolt at 2.30pm in a nice little

Premiere 1 jet. Just me. I was meeting Geraldine in Portofino. She was being picked up by the hotel car from Milan, where she's been living. Got to Northolt and was told our slot – that's the time you can take off – had been changed to 3.20pm. Very annoying. When that happens I always get on the plane – on this occasion at 1.45pm – and the pilot puts in a 'ready' signal. Often you get to go on the scheduled time or even earlier. But air traffic control in Brussels weren't having any of it. They asked if the pilot wanted to withdraw his flight plan and put in another one for an earlier departure. That's dangerous because you can wait a couple of hours if you're unlucky. Eventually took off at 3.20pm. Please note the traumas the rich have to live with. In order to pass the time I had three packets of Walker's crisps ready salted, not flavoured, and a pack of Smarties. This is not totally advisable for a diet. From Genoa (that's where you land for Portofino) we drove to the Hotel Splendido. A very beautiful setting. I recommend it. Dinner there was melon (delicious), which I was told came from 80 miles east of Portofino, some crisp Italian bread called galetta and then fried scampi with fried zucchini. Then a lemon sorbet and some petit four biscuits. There were some scales in the bathroom. They were that annoying type with a lever wobbling about so it's difficult to see your exact weight. I didn't dare weigh myself at night anyway in case I got depressed. Leave it to the morning, I thought.

THURSDAY 29 JUNE
Morning weight 81.7kg or 12st 12lbs. An increase of half a pound. Not too ghastly. Breakfast on the terrace

overlooking a marvellous hill with a castle on. Hillsides all around with only a few old villas and the sea and the harbour of Portofino. One of the great views. Breakfast: a croissant, some other bit of bread, marmalade, butter, orange juice, a cappuccino. When I tried the marmalade, I said to Geraldine, 'This marmalade is not as good as the cheapest marmalade I bought in Waitrose when I was buying on a pensioner's money for the day.' She said, 'Well, it's apricot jam, not marmalade.' I said, 'I thought it didn't taste very orangey.' So I opened the marmalade jar and that's how I had an extra bread roll. Except it wasn't a bread roll. It was some kind of bubbly-surfaced Italian bread. Very good, too. They cleared a terrace for Geraldine and me overlooking the incredible view. Very refreshing. She does crosswords and occasionally I supply an answer. Or she reads. I think about life. Lunch at the restaurant down by the pool: galetta crispbread, still mineral water with fresh lemon juice added, spaghetti with cherry tomatoes and basil (very good), half a melon, wild strawberries and three very good home-made biscuits. It's very hot. I shouldn't have had spaghetti really. But there's no point in being in Italy and not eating the local food. We dieters may put on a bit of weight. What's needed is the willpower to pull it back if it gets serious. I told Geraldine a story about spaghetti. When I was making a film called *Lawman* in Durango, Mexico, the star was my dearest friend ever in showbusiness, Burt Lancaster. He had a terrible temper – grabbed me by the throat and threatened to kill me at least twice. But so what? Anyway, Burt had a big caravan in the dusty desert town near our Western Street location. He played a fanatical sheriff. Burt was brought up in Little Italy in New York, so he loved spaghetti. He used to make it every lunchtime in his caravan. His personal staff, make-up, driver and voice coach would eat it with him. I sat in a special tent with the two other 'above the line' stars – that's actors whose names go above the title. They were two of the Hollywood greats – Robert Ryan and Lee J Cobb. We had special food, still from the Mexican caterer, but better than the crew and other actors, who ate in a big marquee. One of the other actors was Robert Duvall, at the time unknown. He never stopped complaining to his agent that the stars and I got better food than he did! One lunchtime Robert Ryan, Lee J Cobb and I had finished our lunch (lamb chops, veggies and a pudding and coffee) when into our tent walked Burt Lancaster with an enormous bowl of spaghetti. 'I've just made this spaghetti for you, Robert,' said Burt, with a smile that often had a hint of menace. None of us dared say we'd already eaten. 'Thank you, Burt,' said Bob Ryan. And Burt gave him an enormous portion. Then he gave Lee J Cobb some and then me. 'It's great, you'll love it,' said Burt as he went back to his air-conditioned caravan. 'We'll have to eat it,' I said. 'If Burt sees we've left it he'll be impossible for days!' So the three of us somehow or other ate this spaghetti on top of everything else we'd eaten. Whenever I get spaghetti I think of that boiling hot day in the Mexican sun in the outlands of Durango. Around 6.30pm I walked with the hotel's gem, Fausto Allegri, and Geraldine down the hill to Portofino and back up. This is quite strenuous. Fausto knows everyone in Portofino. Who is doing what to whom. He also knows everything about the hotel and what strange and wonderful things are going on there. He plays the cheerful buffoon. But beneath it is great knowledge and steel. He was a legendary concierge. They now call him Guest Relations Manager. He used to have long white hair, like an out-of-work violinist, but he's trimmed it a bit. Every morning he bends down and I put my hand on his head, blessing him as if I was the Pope. I'm sure you do that to hotel staff when you go away. Doesn't everybody? Dinner at the Splendido on a wonderful table – what the Americans call 'by the rail' – overlooking one of the greatest views in the world as day turns to night. The freebie starter was fish soup with rosemary. Then lobster and prawn salad dressed with rosemary and olive oil. This was an attempt at diet as it's a starter course. Then – which I shouldn't have had – apple and plum strudel flavoured with cinnamon and served with green apple sorbet. Finally, mint tea. An absolutely delicious dinner. But far too much eaten today. Night weight on hotel scales 83kg.

FRIDAY 30 JUNE
Morning weight 81.7kg or 12st 12lbs. No increase from yesterday, but half a pound up from Wednesday! Either the scales are wrong or problems will show up later. Breakfast: croissant, other bread thing, butter, marmalade, cappuccino, orange juice. Lunch by pool: this galetta crispbread, which is made down the coast in nearby Santa Margherita, as is the rest of the bread they serve at the Splendido. Same spaghetti as yesterday. A few bits of fish from the buffet (one tiny bit fried!). Fausto says I should

put olive oil on my spaghetti. I'm resisting. Then an apple sorbet and some biscuits. At 6.30pm we went on a hefty walk right up the hill on the other side of the harbour to a castle. On the way down into the lovely harbour, Fausto recommended I have some ice cream at an exterior café called Gelateria San Giorgio, recently bought by the Splendido hotel. I had a vanilla and a pistachio. It was the worst ice cream I've ever eaten! Appalling. Fausto, I noticed, having recommended the ice cream, ordered only a Bellini, as did Geraldine. The Bellinis were very good. That's champagne and fresh peach juice. Some of the best ice cream in the world is at Mikki in Santa Margherita, only 10 minutes away. I suggested to Carlo, the food and beverage manager for the Splendido – who is in charge of the gelateria as well – that he spend at least two weeks in Mikki learning about ice cream. That's me, you see, always trying to be helpful. Dinner was at a restaurant in the harbour called Puny. Puny's real name is Luigi Miroli. Italy's lovable ex-prime minister, Silvio Berlusconi, who has a villa nearby, is frequently in Puny. Indeed, when he won the last election he won, he was photographed the next day in the square of Portofino with his arms round Mr Puny. I think the food is fantastic. I had sliced capone fish with shrimps. Now they tell me the fish is called zaranella. It's a white local fish cooked slice by slice with vegetables, accompanied by scampi with a green sauce made from parsley, capers, anchovies, garlic and olive oil. The waiter said it was an old recipe from the ships. Then I had pappardelle with basil and tomato. Then moscardini, which are tiny, freshly caught, local octopus, with rosemary and lemon and some boiled potatoes. Then mixed fruit, fried cream (yes, I did say fried cream), a pear and fried almonds. Lovely. Diet food? No! I didn't dare weigh myself that night!

SATURDAY 1 JULY
Morning weight 81.7kg or 12st 12lbs. I find this odd. No increase. But I checked many times and that's what the scales said! Breakfast: croissant, more bread, jam, orange juice. Took a one-hour speedboat trip to Vernazza. An enchanting little village, part of what is called Cinque Terra, five such places hugging the Mediterranean with high cliffs behind them. Vernazza is totally unspoiled and beautiful. Here there is an ordinary place called Trattoria Gianni Franzi. But ordinary it isn't! As an example, it is where Lady Ruth Rogers, co-chef and co-owner of the famous River Café, comes to learn about Italian cooking in Gianni's kitchen. It's where she had the 21st birthday party for her son. Since the River Café is not only the best Italian food in London, but overall the best food in London, you'd better believe Gianni knows a thing or two. I had flat black spaghetti with a lightly curried scampi sauce. This was preceded by a mixed appetiser of anchovy and octopus in many styles. Dessert was a lemon granita with vodka. A rather good little band appeared in the square. They were all old men but extremely proficient and cheerful. They had their own amplifier. Two guitars, clarinet, double bass and tambourines. The lady collecting for them went to the next café but not to ours and I had 10 Euros ready for them. I thought they looked like Americans. Gianni said he thought they were Romanian! Dinner was back at the

Splendido. I had melon, then fried scampi with fried zucchini, a Bellini and, for dessert, an apple and lemon sorbet and some biscuits.

SUNDAY 2 JULY
Morning weight 81.7kg or 12st 12lbs. Continental breakfast of croissant, orange juice, coffee. Lunch by the pool: galetta crispbread, spaghetti with cherry tomato and basil, apple sorbet with wild strawberries. Dinner at Puny in the harbour of Portofino. Definitely one of my favourite restaurants in the world. I had shrimps Maron and little octopus that had been in the sea an hour earlier for a starter. Also a slice of grilled fish, which Puny tells me was cooked in the oven for one minute. Then spaghetti with anchovies and rocket. Main course, shrimps with rosemary and lemon. Dessert, a vanilla semifreddo with strawberries and sauce. One of the great meals. Lovely view of the harbour and the square, and the castle on the hill opposite.

MONDAY 3 JULY
Morning weight 82.5kg or 13st. Going up, but still in my current (but later to change) OK zone. Breakfast: croissant, butter, jam, orange juice, coffee. Lunch by pool: melon (for the first time verging on the soft!), then spaghetti with tomato and basil, a Bellini and wild strawberries for dessert. In the evening I went on Sir Donald Gosling's enormous – and I do mean enormous – boat. Crew of 27 people. It was rented out. Michael and Shakira Caine were guests of Jerry Perencio and his wife. He has a large number of Spanish-speaking TV and radio stations in

America as well as presenting concerts by Pavarotti and other major stars. Also with us was a man called Michael, head of Herbal Life, a big US health food company. A very few canapés there before going to the Splendido for dinner. As host I was a beacon of moderation. I had melon, ravioli, and a lemon and apple sorbet.

TUESDAY 4 JULY
Morning weight 83.7kg or 13st 2½lbs. Getting into disaster. But if you read on you'll see how your hero (me!) not only took it all off but settled on a new 'proper' weight of 12 stone three pounds. So however wrong you go, with willpower you can change your mistakes! Usual breakfast of croissant, jam, butter, orange juice, coffee. Lunch by pool: spaghetti with tomatoes, wild strawberries, lemon sorbet, biscuits. For dinner Fausto recommended – and came with us to – O Magazin. This is a restaurant further down the port in Portofino, by bobbing boats. It's out of the activity of the square. Fausto had often recommended total duds. But this was a triumph. I'd been to Portofino many times and never tried this place. It's great. The house appetiser was five kinds of fish, including octopus, and some potato. Then we had a selection of various pastas with shrimp and walnut sauce. Main course was local grilled prawns from Santa Margherita. I had ice cream, which wasn't brilliant. Tasted a bit like Wall's, which I quite like. And wild strawberries. I tried a tiny bit of Fausto's apple cake too.

WEDNESDAY 5 JULY

Morning weight 84kg or 13st 3lbs. Breakfast: croissant, other bread, jam, orange juice. Lunch by the pool: half a melon, cold fish and veg from the buffet and, foolishly, two scoops of vanilla ice cream plus one scoop of pistachio ice cream and some biscuits. On the private jet back I had a few Smarties. I'd have eaten the whole packet but Geraldine wrested them from me. Then after dinner she made me walk for an hour in Holland Park. It was her birthday, bless her. You'd think she might have loosened up a bit. Dinner: back to the sheep's milk yoghurt, 200g, with raspberries and jam. Night weight 84.7kg. Note I didn't dare record night weight in the hotel. It would have been too depressing. Kept me awake!

THURSDAY 6 JULY

Morning weight 83.7kg or 13st 2½lbs. An increase of five pounds in Italy. Not great, but not as dreadful as I feared after knocking back a daily diet of spaghetti, other pasta, ice cream and God knows what else plus croissants for breakfast. Still five pounds up in seven days shows how easy it is to be remodelled as the original fat pig. Now the familiar breakfast of 200g sheep's milk yoghurt plus jam plus clementine juice. 11-ish: coffee with single malt 1977 Macallan Scotch whisky bunged in. Lunch: roast chicken leg, carrots, Brussels sprouts. In the early evening I went to make a speech in the park in a marquee by the Albert Memorial. It was for the Royal Parks people, who were inaugurating some new policy for filming in the Royal Parks. Mark Camley, the Royal Parks boss, agreed I should check with the Queen about wanting to be buried on Cambridge Green, which is part of St James's Park and where my National Police Memorial is. He had no objection. Well, there are some dogs buried in Hyde Park. Surely I qualify as equal to a dog! Maybe not. I drank nothing and avoided the canapés. Went home after and had 400g of sheep's milk yoghurt in two servings, jam with each, and some raspberries and other berries. Geraldine forced me to do a one-hour walk in Holland Park. During the day I had a few pieces of Rococo sugar-free and dairy-free chocolate. Night weight 82.7kg.

FRIDAY 7 JULY

Morning weight 82.7kg or 13st ¼lb. This is unbelievable. It has never, ever happened before. It seems I lost no weight overnight at all! I know my night weight yesterday was accurate because I checked it twice and thought, 'That's good, I'll be well below 13 stone tomorrow!' But it's exactly the same! Normally it's at least a pound lighter. Am I turning into some monster from outer space? Is my body undergoing drastic change? Let's see what happens tonight. Either way, it's a good result, to lose two and three-quarter pounds in two days. It shows, and please read carefully and do it yourself, that if you get a bit overweight, deal with it drastically and at once. Don't let it slip on, as I've done dozens of times before, and blow up to your old size or worse. Breakfast: 200g sheep's milk yoghurt, jam, clementine juice. 11-ish: coffee with single malt Scotch. Lunch: grilled salmon with fresh peas, fruit salad and cream. Dessert was because we had a guest, the Honourable

Camilla Jessel. Very posh. Known her since she was 17. Daren't say more, she may sue. Very nice person. Around 4pm: iced coffee with the 1977 single malt Scotch. Dinner: a bit of melon, which was hard and horrible. I'd been having these marvellous melons in Italy. I come home and my cook leaves me this rubbish melon in the fruit bowl. I shall make my feelings known. So I had some smoked salmon from Lidgate, normally a first-class butcher, but that wasn't much good either! A bit of Philadelphia cream cheese, tiny bit of avocado (that was tough!) followed by lamb's milk yoghurt with jam and raspberries. That's reliable. Then walked for an hour in Holland Park with Geraldine. Should be a slimming day. We'll see. Night weight 83.5kg.

SATURDAY 8 JULY
Morning weight 82.7kg or 13st ¼lb. No change from yesterday morning. Odd. I expected to be down a bit. Breakfast: 200g organic live sheep's milk yoghurt, jam, clementine juice. Lunch at San Lorenzo, a much under-rated restaurant brilliantly and very personally run by Mara Berni, who keeps falling down the stairs. I told her to go down stairs as I do, holding on and slowly. I demonstrated. She'll take no notice. She's been running the place for 43 years. It's still marvellous. Mara knows everyone and greets them like it's her home. Unfortunately she uses that as a reason not to let me pay. I left £100 on the table years ago and Mara chased me down Beauchamp Place, forcing me to take it back, saying, 'You can't buy your way in here!' So I gave her presents of quite valuable ornaments from my house,

and flowers and clothes for her grandchildren. I said, 'Mara, soon I'll have no furniture left. You'll have the three-piece suite and the telly. Please let me pay!' She wouldn't. So now I give the waiter £50 surreptitiously as I leave. This time I ate a bit of bread and butter, Buck's Fizz, asparagus (no sauce), an incredibly good shrimp risotto with organic rice, and the best chocolate ice cream you could hope to have. This was an outstanding meal. I shall not be eating anything remotely substantial later. Before dinner I drank some strange vegetable drink made from fresh veggies at Luscious Organic, my local ever-so-healthy food place and café. Geraldine got it and brought it back. It was green, no great taste, but you knew it was good for you. Then went to see *Hay Fever* with Judi Dench at the Theatre Royal Haymarket. Old-fashioned, very funny in some places, deadly dull in others. The Ritz hotel had parked my car so as it's next to The Wolseley I went in there on my way back. That was a mistake. Had a vanilla milkshake. Very good taste, bit thin in texture, straw much too thin and too short. Some white bread roll and butter and then a foie gras cum pâté thing with brioche. All this around 10pm. Far too late to eat if you don't absolutely have to. Particularly if you're on a diet. Night weight 83.1kg.

SUNDAY 9 JULY
Morning weight 82.4kg or 12st 13¾lbs. Good, I'm back below 13 stone. That's always consoling. Breakfast: sheep's milk yoghurt with jam and orange juice. For lunch I was going to go to the Petersham Nurseries Café, which is good. But yesterday, for the first time, I spoke to

their restaurant manager, Rachel Lewis. I thought she was so unwelcoming, horrid and generally snooty that I cancelled the table and booked at the River Café instead. That is always superb. Lady Ruth Rogers, the co-owner, was cooking. I said, 'You ignored me in Vernazza last week. Gianni Franzi said you were staying there and you'd come down to see me, but you didn't!' Lady Rogers said, 'I wasn't there! I haven't been to Vernazza for months.' This was very odd because if you go back to 1 July you'll see Gianna spoke of Lady Rogers most clearly. I believe Her Ladyship's version totally. Then a lovely young woman came over whom I didn't recognise (because I'm really stupid and never recognise anyone). It was Jemima Khan, there with Hugh Grant. Both very nice people. They were at the next table. Food was, as always, terrific. I had crushed strawberry juice with prosecco, some toasted bruschetta with olive oil, pappardelle with mushrooms and pigeon from Anjou. (I don't know why all the good pigeons are announced on menus as coming from Anjou. I've never seen one that reads, 'Pigeon from Michael Winner's Garden'. Why?) I finished with a very good strawberry sorbet and fresh mint tea. I also nicked a bit of Geraldine's incredible Chocolate Nemesis, which is a sort of rich chocolate cream cake. A senior person in the restaurant game was there. When I said I'd had a conversation with Rachel Lewis at the Petersham Nurseries Café that was considerably less than welcoming, this person responded, 'She's not very charming, is she?' I prevented myself from exploding into my real view because I'm so discreet and delicate. Early evening walk in Holland Park after a modest dinner of whooshed-about vegetables made into a green juice, plus sheep's milk yoghurt with strawberries and jam. This should be a thinning day, although lunch was quite heavy all in all. Night weight 83.3kg.

MONDAY 10 JULY

Morning weight 82.7kg or 13st ¼lb. Tiny increase, oh dear. Breakfast: sheep's milk yoghurt, jam, clementine juice. 11-ish: coffee with 1977 Macallan single malt whisky bunged in plus brown crystal sugar. Small piece of Rococo chocolate. Lunch: grilled Dover sole, carrots, peas. Visit from Chris Rea and his wife, Joan (he a famous singer, they my favourite people). They had a cuppa tea. Before dinner some Dom Perignon champagne and nuts and raisins. Dinner at Le Caprice with Geraldine and my assistant Dinah. I had a piece of white roll and butter. Duck salad. 50 grams Golden Oscietra caviar, which wasn't gold at all, with some crème fraîche and two small blinis. Mineral water. Night weight 82.8kg.

TUESDAY 11 JULY

Morning weight 82.2kg or 12st 13¼lbs. Nice little decrease there. I'd like you to know the agony I go through just to tell you my weight. I first weighed myself at 6.30am, three times. On each occasion my weight was 82kg. Five minutes later I weighed myself again on the same scales. I had eaten and drunk nothing in between. This time my weight showed as 82.3kg, for four times on and off the scales. The fifth time I went on the scales, just a second later, my weight showed 82.5kg! It held at that for three more consecutive 'weigh-ins'! Then I did a bit of gardening. Ate and drank nothing. Came back at 7.45am and weighed myself again. Now the weight was 82.2kg. It held at that for four more visits to the scales. So that's the weight I've put down. Nobody said life was easy! But we ex-fat pigs, determined not to slip back to obesity and gluttony, go through all this with pleasure. Because when we look in the mirror we can see the difference! Breakfast: sheep's milk yoghurt, jam, clementine juice. 11-ish: coffee with single malt Macallan 1977 Scotch whisky in it and two teaspoonfuls of brown crystal sugar. I hope you're noting that I've been eating cakes, sugar, white bread and butter, nuts, ice cream – all the things normal diets tell you to avoid. Moderation. That's the word. If you splash out – extra moderation. This diary proves dieting is possible without serious mental damage. And you know, when you eat in moderation as a matter of course, the pain diminishes. It becomes a manageable way of life. If you haven't decided by now that you can do it, and more importantly that you will, you're a pathetic, stupid lost cause – as I was for 70 years. But remember that while there's life, there's hope! Lunch: a whole cold lobster, bit of mayonnaise, some salad. Lobster, I'm assured, isn't fattening. But I felt a bit full after eating it. Held back on the Hellmann's mayonnaise. Around 4pm: an iced coffee with single malt Scotch and white sugar! Dinner: 200g sheep's milk yoghurt, raspberries, brown granulated sugar. Vegetable drink. Then went with Geraldine for a walk in Holland Park. Put on my little trainers and everything! Did not walk at great speed though. Night weight 82.8kg.

WEDNESDAY 12 JULY

Morning weight 82.1kg or 12st 13lbs. Breakfast: 200g sheep's milk yoghurt (I put strawberry jam in it), clementine juice. 11-ish: coffee with single malt Scotch, crystal brown sugar. Lunch: grilled plaice, green beans, corn on the cob off the cob, if you get my meaning. 4-ish: coffee with single malt Scotch. Occasionally Rococo sugar-free and dairy-free chocolate. Pre-dinner: my vegetable drink plus some nuts and raisins, on the balcony overlooking my large garden with many mature trees. Flowers galore. We have not suffered from the hosepipe ban because I have men watering from cans and large plastic containers on wheels. Many men for many hours. Just costs rather a lot. Dinner: grilled fillet steak, raspberries. Afterwards a walk in Holland Park. Met my over-the-road neighbour, lyricist Don Black (*Born Free*, *Diamonds Are Forever* and other hits). He tells me the large premises on the corner of my road and Kensington High Street, which have been empty for a couple of years, are going to be a gymnasium. They were going to be a restaurant. I met the man who was opening it. He showed me around all his kitchen equipment and everything. Unfortunately he hadn't got a restaurant licence, and the people in the posh apartment block that the premises are part of objected. So he was lumbered with second-hand kitchen equipment and empty premises! I bet he's glad someone has at last taken them. It's a funny area, this western end of Kensington High Street. Used to be very genteel. Bebe Daniels, who was a US movie star and British radio star, had an antique shop here. She was married to another old-time Hollywood star, Ben Lyon, who was the lead in Howard Hughes' *Hell's Angels*. Then there were two lovely old ladies with a dress shop. Three well-dressed muggers came in broad daylight, locked the shop, forced them into a changing booth and robbed them of everything. So they retired. Now it's a mish-mash. Asian mini-market, bicycle shop, charity shop, newsagent. Not as classy as it was when I moved to my house in 1946. But then, neither am I. Before bed I made a hot chocolate drink with some brown crystal sugar in it. Night weight 82.7kg.

THURSDAY 13 JULY
Morning weight 81.4kg or 12st 11½lbs. I'm rather pleased with that. It's one of my lowest weights since I started dieting. It's also an unusually large weight loss overnight. We ex-fat pigs notice these things. Breakfast: sheep's milk yoghurt, jam, clementine juice. 11-ish: coffee with single malt Scotch. Lunch at The Wolseley with Paola. That brilliant actor and nice person Bill Nighy was at the next table. Half a white bread roll with butter, Buck's Fizz, roast suckling pig with extra crackling, potato balls (I think they're kind of mashed and fried), a summer pudding with clotted cream and some of Paola's strawberry tart and ice cream. Fresh mint tea. Not a slimming meal. But from time to time these things are okay. 4-ish: coffee with Scotch and crystal brown sugar. Dinner: 200g sheep's milk yoghurt and raspberries. Then Geraldine and I went to some reception for a new restaurant Gordon Ramsay is opening in Sloane Street. It was previously called Pengelley's and was bloody awful. I'm not surprised it closed. Gordon told me he lost a

million pounds on it! I resisted the canapés but did take one very small marshmallow thing. Also they gave me some freshly squeezed orange juice. I hope the place does well. I like Gordon and his wife Tana. Then it became, for me, a very late night because at 11pm I had to report to *This Week*, Andrew Neil's TV programme, to be in a piece about explosive rudeness following Zidane head-butting some Italian in the World Cup football. Andrew referred to me as 'the rudest man in England', which is total nonsense, but who cares! I didn't get home until 12.30am. Dazed, I forgot to weigh myself!

FRIDAY 14 JULY
Morning weight 81.4kg or 12st 11¼lbs. Same as yesterday. That's good in view of my excessive lunch. But it shows that if you don't eat much in the evening you can still be in good shape. Breakfast: sheep's milk yoghurt, jam, clementine juice. 11-ish: coffee with Scotch. Lunch: grilled salmon, peas and asparagus. 4-ish: iced coffee with Scotch. Pre-dinner: nuts and raisins with a vegetable drink. Dinner: smoked salmon and Philadelphia cream cheese sandwich on brown bread, an apple. Walked for over an hour, including a trip to Geraldine's new flat 15 minutes away. Did some garden watering. Night weight – forgot to take it!

SATURDAY 15 JULY
Morning weight 81kg or 12st 10½lbs. I congratulate myself! That's very good! Breakfast: sheep's milk live organic yoghurt with marmalade chucked in, clementine juice. 11-ish: coffee with sugar and single malt Scotch. I

was told a story this morning by a friend who phoned me about a charity auction at a 'do' he organised. One of the prizes was dinner cooked at home by a very famous British chef. It was bought for £48,000 by the head of a well-known bank. The chef attended the house and discussed the menu and the arrangements. Come the day the banker, an American, had asked people from New York and from Europe, and they all came over. Which is more than the chef did! He never turned up. Never wrote, never telephoned, just didn't show! 'We had to give him the £48,000 back,' said my friend ruefully. Knowing the chef well I was not surprised at all! Lunch at The Wolseley: bit of roll and butter, Buck's Fizz, potted shrimps, endive, walnut and Roquefort cheese salad and, for dessert, vanilla ice cream with chocolate sauce. Bit strong. So for dinner just some nuts and raisins and my liquidised vegetable juice from Luscious Organic in Kensington High Street. Then went to the Royal Court Theatre to see Tom Stoppard's play *Rock "N" Roll*. Met a couple at the theatre who were very big in 1960s – Victor Lowndes, who was head of *Playboy* in the UK, and his wife Marilyn Cole, who was Britain's first *Playboy* centrefold. They're both lovely people, very respectable. As we chatted on the pavement in the interval I eventually said, 'Don't you notice I've lost nearly three stone?' 'You look like I remember you,' said Marilyn. Victor said the same. We'd seen each other so little since I ballooned into fat piggy-Winner they didn't even realise my immense achievement. Oh well. Before bed a feeble attempt at an iced chocolate drink. Didn't work because without staff (cook's day off), no ice available in my bedroom kitchen and I couldn't be bothered to walk downstairs! Night weight 81.4kg.

SUNDAY 16 JULY
Morning weight 80.9kg or 12st 10¼lbs. This shows you can eat a pig-lunch and still lose weight if you really keep it down in the evening. Breakfast: sheep's milk yoghurt, jam, orange juice. To Michael Caine's house in Surrey for lunch. Brilliant as usual. A Pimms, then salmon, new potatoes, courgettes, peas, asparagus, ice cream, rhubarb from Michael's garden. On to the tail end of an 80th birthday lunch party for an old movie friend in Holland Park. There was Rita Tushingham and, of all people, the very lively Mandy Rice-Davies. While her old-time pal Christine Keeler rots in some ghastly council flat, Mandy has done very well. She told me she now lives on the Wentworth Estate. All mansions, some of the poshest in England. Good for her! Dinner: my freshly made veggie drink, nuts and raisins. Walk in Holland Park. Then watched Spielberg's *War of the Worlds* in my private cinema. Shows even Spielberg can't get it right all the time. Just before bed three chocolate biscuits! Night weight 80.9kg.

MONDAY 17 JULY
Morning weight 80.3kg or 12st 9lbs. Very good! I don't quite see how I lost one and a quarter pounds, with what I ate yesterday, but that's what the scales told me! I'm over three stone less than I used to be! Breakfast: sheep's milk yoghurt with marmalade in it, clementine juice. 11-ish: iced coffee with organic milk, white sugar, single

malt Scotch. Lunch: grilled Dover sole, carrots, peas. In the afternoon my assistant Dinah went into the attic to look at old suitcases full of shirts. I'd already given a lot from there to her husband. Those I could now get into. I'm wearing quite a few shirts from my 'Maybe one day' cupboard. Although I've had jackets taken in, most of my shirts are very big for the new slimline Winner. She brought some very good shirts down but sadly the stomach I have left, although a shadow of its former self, still protruded too much for these to be done up. I told her to keep them in the attic. Who knows, one day I might be thin enough to wear them! She is now going to look in the attic area behind my dressing room as opposed to the enormous attic at the top of the house. Maybe that'll reveal something. (Sadly, it didn't!) After a glass of Château Lafite 1985 at home, I went to Scalini for dinner. Total disaster. Bit of bread, couple of cubes of Parmesan, bowl of fresh tomatoes in olive oil, three spare ribs, many too many slices of fried zucchini and then, to screw it all up, a large zabaglione, which is a sort of sugar-full cream custard made with raw eggs and other things, plus one half of the rich biscuit accompanying it. The brief walk around the block when I got home didn't do much. Misjudged the garage door entrance and bashed the Suzuki front wing and bumper into the side of it! What a moron! And the only alcohol I'd had at dinner was one small limoncello liqueur. Night weight – forgot to take it. 'You forgot to take it on 13 July as well!' I hear you say. Too bad. Nobody's perfect and you can't get your money back.

TUESDAY 18 JULY

Morning weight 80.8kg or 12st 10lbs. That biggish dinner put me up one pound. So if you're on your diet, and I hope you've started it by now, it's OK to have a biggie-dinnie from time to time. But pull back afterwards. Watch what I eat today! Breakfast: the usual sheep's milk yoghurt, jam, clementine juice. 11-ish: coffee with Macallan single malt Scotch. 12-ish: some Rococo dairy-free, sugar-free chocolate. Note the word 'some' means more than 'a little' – in this case about seven small squares. Someone said to me recently, 'Are you putting the amounts you eat in your diet book?' I replied, 'I'm not taking a scales to every restaurant and weighing the amount of each item on the plate. I'm kind of indicating it.' The questioner looked very snippy at that. Bloody cheek! Lunch: crabmeat, bit of Hellmann's mayonnaise, bit of salad. PM: bit of Rococo chocolate. No coffee with Scotch! Dinner: vegetable drink, salted peanuts and raisins. This is the sort of thing you have to do if you want to lose weight. Walk in Holland Park. We saw Dame Shirley Porter, the disgraced ex-leader of West-minster Council, walk by. She was extremely unhelpful when I wanted to put up my first police memorial, to WPC Yvonne Fletcher, in St James's Square. After waiting forever and getting no decision from the West-minster Council I rang Dame Shirley at home and said, 'Could we please have permission to honour this young lady?' She said, 'What's the deal?' Unbelievable that! I thought, 'If she wants a deal, if she thinks we're trading in scrap metal, I'll give her one.' 'I'll make the memorial six inches deep instead of nine,' I offered. That did it. We got our permission! When the memorial was unveiled by Margaret Thatcher, with all other political leaders – Neil Kinnock, David Owen, David Steel – in attendance, Shirley Porter, the leader of the council for the borough where Yvonne gave her life, didn't even bother to turn up! I did not greet her in Holland Park. She did not greet me! What a cow! Night weight 81kg.

WEDNESDAY 19 JULY

Morning weight 79.9kg or 12st 8lbs. Getting very low! Will I have to have 68 jackets taken in yet again? Being below my safety weight zone is good. Particularly as I'm off to Venice next week, which could be fattening. Always best to go on holiday with a few pounds in hand. Breakfast: sheep's milk yoghurt, jam, clementine juice. 11-ish: coffee with single malt Scotch, brown crystal sugar. Lunch: grilled salmon with rich hollandaise sauce, broad beans, asparagus. Gael Boglione, the terribly nice owner of the Petersham Nurseries Café, rang me to apologise for the grotesquely unwelcoming behaviour of her restaurant manager when I phoned to make a reservation on Saturday 8 July. 'She wanted to phone herself to apologise,' said Gael. 'You mean she read about it in the *Sunday Times*. Everyone's talking about it, so she considered apologising!' I said. 'Not quite the same as realising you did something silly and phoning a few hours after the event!' Funnily enough I expected lots of letters attacking me about this. Instead I got hardly any – yet quite a lot saying the staff at the Petersham Nurseries Café were sniffy and rude! Whenever I write attacking some ill-performing restaurant staff member I always wonder if I might have been wrong. And always, without fail, readers write in and say they suffered from the same sort of behaviour from the same person. Some, of course, attack me! Good, that's part of the fun! Dinner: nuts, raisins, vegetable drink. Then a walk in Battersea Park. Learn from this. If you don't have to go out where the temptations are great, it is not necessary to eat a big dinner at home. You can eat healthily but sparsely, as I have done for the last two nights. I had an iced chocolate drink with sugar added to finish the evening. Night weight 80kg.

THURSDAY 20 JULY

Morning weight 79.6kg or 12st 7½lbs. Oh my gawd! Another half pound down! Over half a stone lost in the two weeks since 6 July! I am now three stone two and a half pounds less than I used to be! And it's all been quite painless. Believe me, you can do this too. Breakfast: sheep's milk yoghurt, jam, clementine juice. 11-ish: coffee with single malt Scotch. Lunch: cold lobster and salad. My alterations tailor, Michael, came with eight more jackets he'd taken in and was given a further six. I also gave him one shirt. He said he'd charge £15 a shirt to diminish their size for me. I have 226 shirts. So at £15 each that'd be £3,390. 'Is it worth it?' I ask myself. So far I haven't decided! Dinner: a fillet steak, which I grilled myself. Left it in a bit too long. I always slice steaks, so you have to watch very closely. Still, it was okay. Should have been historic. Also had my veggie drink plus four chocolate biscuits and, later, an iced chocolate before bed. Walked in Holland Park. Night weight 80kg.

FRIDAY 21 JULY

Morning weight 79.3kg or 12st 6¾lbs. I am wasting away! Another three-quarters of a pound gone! I'm completely off the chart I made showing kilograms and stones and pounds. I've increased this chart downwards many times. Before today it only went down to 79.4 kilograms, which is 12 stone seven pounds. Now I've had to add many more downward weight situations. May this joy be yours! Breakfast: sheep's milk yoghurt, jam, clementine juice. 11-ish: coffee with single malt Scotch. Lunch: rather small grilled sole, corn off the cob, fresh peas, a blob of butter. After lunch, a bit of Rococo dairy-free and sugar-free chocolate. 4pm: tried the new coconut-flavoured Actimel. All right, not historic, but nicer than the normal one. Dinner at La Noisette, a newly opened, Gordon Ramsay-owned place in Sloane Street. Very posh menu. I had what was laughingly known as 'Summer Favourites' – five courses excluding dessert! They were small courses but mercifully came very quickly. I started with very good bread, then a Buck's Fizz. Then almond gazpacho; smoked paprika, shrimp and tomato sorbet (see what I mean by posh?!); Berkshire crayfish, girolles and herb velouté; then watermelon carpaccio, goat's milk feta and rocket; then wild trout with English peas, beurre rouge and mustard emulsion; then the main course of saddle of Lincolnshire rabbit, snails, squid and bean salad. Get that! It was very good and as every course was so tiny it wasn't that filling. Then I had the 'classic dessert', which changes every day. That night it was some sort of cherry flan with ice cream. This'll put weight on, I thought. Night weight 80.1kg.

SATURDAY 22 JULY
Morning weight (amazingly down!) 79.2kg or 12st 6½lbs.
An odd day. I was due to go to the wedding of Anji
Hunter, ex-aide to Tony Blair, and the Sky political
correspondent Adam Boulton at 1pm at a church in
Piccadilly, followed a reception at Spencer House, which
was just canapés, drinks and speeches. So breakfast as
usual: sheep's milk yoghurt, jam, clementine juice. Then
at 11.30am I had two slices of brown toast with
marmalade and jam and Philadelphia cream cheese, and
a cup of coffee with single malt Scotch in it. Then we
went off to the church. Except we missed the ceremony
because all of central London was closed off for a
Palestinian march against the Israelis going into
Lebanon, among other things. It took me two hours to be
driven the three miles from my house to the church. By
the time we got there everyone had more or less left. I
went inside to see the flower decoration and then on to
Spencer House. There I asked Tony Blair (whom I know
and like), 'On a scale of one to ten, how happy have you
been the last year?' This is a Marlon Brando question.
Tony thought for a second and said, 'Seven.' 'That's very
good,' I said, 'considering all the stick you're taking.' 'I'm
doing what I like doing,' responded Tone. 'When I first
met you, when you'd just become Labour leader, you
answered four,' I said, 'so that's a good increase!' David
Blunkett, ex-Home Secretary, was there with dog. When
I said, 'Hello, David, Michael Winner,' he said, 'Nice to
see you.' When I introduced Geraldine he said, 'Nice
to see you' to her! As he's blind, I found that odd. I only
ate two or three canapés at most. Only drank water. We

left around five and went to the nearby Wolseley for sort of high tea. Earl Grey to be precise. And a tomato omelette, three small sandwiches and a lemon and a lime sorbet. Very nice, too. Later at home, around 10.30pm, I got a bit peckish so I had two freshly squeezed oranges and some nuts and raisins. Night weight 80kg.

SUNDAY 23 JULY
Morning weight 79.3kg or 12st 6¾lbs. Not bad, only a quarter of a pound increase. We're going down to Sir Michael Caine's for lunch today. That'll test the diet. Breakfast: I personally squeezed two oranges for the juice (who says I'm useless in the kitchen!) plus the usual sheep's milk yoghurt and jam. And a small piece of Rococo chocolate. Lunch at the house of Michael and Shakira Caine: the usual superb selection laid out for self-service. Chicken, marvellous boiled potatoes from his garden, beans, cabbage. Very good stuffing. Then superb rhubarb crumble, some sort of cooked peach with cream and Häagen-Dazs toffee ice cream. I took a second helping of that – as all dieters can from time to time. Dinner: one coconut Actimel, a toasted tomato sandwich with olive oil, one glass of fresh veggie extracts. Night weight 80.5kg.

MONDAY 24 JULY
Morning weight 79.3kg or 12st 6¾lbs. Breakfast: sheep's milk yoghurt with jam, clementine juice. Usual coffee with single malt Scotch around 11am. Lunch: grilled salmon, asparagus, carrots. 5pm-ish: iced coffee with sugar. I forgot to put the 1977 Macallan single malt

Scotch in! This is serious. I could die from Scotch deprivation. Dinner: one glass of freshly made veggie extracts, some nuts and raisins. Then a walk in Holland Park. Before bed I went to the kitchen and had two chocolate biscuits! Night weight 79.5kg.

TUESDAY 25 JULY
Morning weight 78.6kg or 12st 5¼lbs. I really am the incredible shrinking man. Another pound and a half bites the dust! It just shows what restraint can do. Mind you, if someone had said to me a year ago I'd be satisfied with a dinner of a glass of vegetable juice and some nuts and raisins, I'd have thought them crazy. But once you get into a different way of life regarding food intake, it is not as painful, and certainly not as difficult, as you might think. It's very simple: when you don't have to eat a lot because you're out or with company, then don't eat a lot. In fact, eat f***ing little! Furthermore you never HAVE to eat a lot, even when you're out. You can still show discipline. Leave a great deal of normal portions on your plate. Breakfast: usual sheep's milk yoghurt, jam, clementine juice. 11-ish: coffee with milk, sugar, single malt Scotch. Lunch: shrimps, salad including avocado, mayonnaise. Dinner: vegetable drink plus nuts and raisins. Walk in Holland Park. I signed a petition organised by some of my neighbours in Abbotsbury Road, around the corner, to prevent a vast O_2 mast going up in a conservation area. I had already helped stop one going on the block of flats near my house, and I helped stop penthouses going onto a period block down the road. I'm also trying to stop the Kensington Council

permitting the destruction of the 1935 Odeon cinema near the junction of my road and the High Street. All this and dieting too. I'm a marvel. Our cinema protests have had some result. The height of the new block was reduced and the original cinema frontage incorporated. Got rather peckish, so just before bed I had a slice of brown bread, one half with butter, the other half with butter and jam! Night weight 78.7kg.

WEDNESDAY 26 JULY
Morning weight 78kg or 12st 4lbs. This is getting ridiculous. I'm now in another weight zone altogether! I'm down a further four pounds in a week! Trousers that were taken in and tight are now wrinkling around the waist. Will everything have to be taken in yet again? Or will I revert to my slim comfort zone of 12 stone 12 pounds to 13 stone two pounds? Breakfast: sheep's milk yoghurt, jam, clementine juice. Lunch: a kipper with ratatouille. On the private jet to Venice I ate a large bag of Kettle chips – 'Sea Salt Crushed with Black Pepper-corns. Hand-cooked. Nothing Artificial'. They were too peppery. Then I had two quarters of bread doubled up as a smoked salmon and cheese sandwich. Then one Ferrero Rocher choccy thing. Then a Fox's glacier mint (two to be precise). I was getting into the holiday spirit. Dinner at Harry's Bar in Venice, my favourite restaurant in all the world. Started with a Bellini – white peach juice and prosecco. The peach juice at Harry's Bar, where the Bellini was invented, is tinned so they can serve the same taste all the year round. It's still great. Then I had chicken croquettes and a croque monsieur (that's sort of toasted,

fried cheese and ham). All very fattening. Then little shrimps from the lagoon, peeled that very morning. Fantastic taste. Then veal ravioli. Then yoghurt ice cream or iced yoghurt, I'm not sure which, and three large bowls of jam were brought, strawberry, prune and orange. I added bits. Finally, mint tea with white sugar. Not a slimming meal! Night weight (now on Cipriani hotel scales) 80kg.

THURSDAY 27 JULY

Morning weight 79kg or 12st 6lbs. Going up already! Had breakfast by the lagoon and the swimming pool. Bowl of mixed berries and cappuccino. Lunch also by the lagoon, although a boat was moored opposite, not helping the view. Parked boats are like parked cars. Hideous. I faxed the manager, Dr Natale Rusconi, from London and the next day the boat was moved. Gone! I ate prosciutto ham and melon, then from the salad bar cherry tomatoes, radishes, onion and various soft cheeses and Parmesan. For dessert, a Bellini sorbet that sat on a bed of sliced peaches. Then an iced cappuccino with bits of chocolate floating in it. At 4.45pm I had a Mentito, which is one of their special cocktails. It's historic. I'll tell you how to make it: 40 grams fresh grapefruit juice, 30 grams fresh lime juice, 15 grams orgeat syrup, lime fruit, brown sugar, fresh mint leaves, crushed ice and soda water. Take half a lime and press with some brown sugar and fresh mint leaves. Fill the glass with crushed ice and soda water. Garnish with lemon, mint and fresh berries. Delicious beyond belief. For dinner I'd been recommended, for the second time in 12 years, the Hotel

Monaco & Grand Canal. The first time was by a strange woman called Lady Rose Lauritzen, who lives in Venice with her very gloomy American husband, an expert on the city who shows US presidents around when they come. This can't be a full-time job, so I guess he spends the rest of the time being miserable. I'd hated the Hotel Monaco & Grand Canal 12 years ago. Now it had been recommended again, this time by a very famous Italian clothes designer, one of those whose name is on his shops all over the world. He, like Lady Lauritzen, said it was where the Venetians went! It has a nice balcony with a marvellous view of the 1630 church of Santa Maria della Salute. There were eight people from Scarborough on one side and four North London Jewish people on the other who spoke a great deal about Marks & Spencer. Venetians I did not see. The food wasn't good. I started with scorpio fish, which turned out to be five bits of white fish, each grilled or cooked with different herbs, none of which made it taste like anything you'd want to eat. This was interspersed with little balls of melon. Then we had some yellow linguine, which was the only really poor pasta I've ever been served in Italy. The main course of white fish cooked in salt that had to be bashed off it was good, but by then I'd given up. So I fled across a little alley to Harry's Bar next door, sat at my usual corner table and ate crêpes, which were fantastic, with vanilla ice cream. I watched the ballet of the waiters serving between the packed tables in the downstairs bar area, which is the only place to be. The owner, Arrigo Cipriani, 75 and elegant, goes around greeting guests and always tells me who everyone is. Mainly Italians. He said, 'The trouble is they used to stay seated but now, because I'm an old banger, a lot of them stand up when I come over.' He is the best. Night weight 80.5kg.

FRIDAY 28 JULY
Morning weight 79.5kg or 12st 7½lbs. This is me ballooning. But luckily I started well below my weight comfort zone. Breakfast: bowl of mixed berries, cappuccino, some grapes, all in a tent. Actually a pavilion. They have two by the pool in the vast gardens that surround it. I pointed them out to Dr Rusconi. 'Why don't I have one of those?' I asked. 'They're privately owned,' he replied. 'Well, the owners aren't there,' I said. I think he was bluffing. Anyway we moved in. They're spectacular. Chairs, air conditioning, a fridge, a bowl of fruit, a deck overlooking the gardens and the pool. Oh, the luxury of it all! Lunch by the lagoon in what I think is one of the best seats in the world. Just beautiful. I had short pasta with tomato, basil and olives. I'd originally ordered a Mentito, but I was talked into having a cocktail that's not on their pretty printed list: half lime with fresh ginger, a strip of cucumber, everything smashed with a little spoon of brown sugar, then they add Angostura bitters, cranberry juice, soda and ginger ale. I also had a white bread roll with green olives in it and, to finish, a Bellini sorbet with fresh peaches, then a Mentito and then a frozen capuccino. Dinner at Harry's Bar. Very dramatic lightning going on. But we got inside before the rain started. I began with Arrigo's bread roll, which is not like any bread you've ever tasted. A Bellini and a tuna tartare with a slightly mustardy sauce. Then lobster

amoricaine with rice pilaf. And a lemon sorbet. This is the best restaurant in the world. No doubt. But not good for dieters!

SATURDAY 29 JULY
Morning weight 80kg or12st 8¼lbs. Like an elevator, I'm going up! But you can do that on my diet as long as you pull back and don't go so far that you're beyond saving. Breakfast by the lagoon: mixed berries and a cappuccino. During the morning a packet of salted peanuts and a Mentito. Very hot! Lunch: a bowl of berries, watermelon, a white bread roll and butter, a scoop of chocolate and vanilla ice cream, three small chocolate biscuit petits fours. The pool area of the Cipriani is a magical place. Lots of trees and flowers and the most enormous, almost Olympic-size pool, very well heated. Dinner at Harry's Bar: rice pilaf with shrimps, mushrooms and peppers. It was called rice pilaf valenciana. Does this mean anything to you? Doesn't to me! David Tang and Anoushka Hempel were there. We met in St Mark's Square afterwards for a drink. I had water! I finished in Harry's Bar with a lemon sorbet.

SUNDAY 30 JULY
Morning weight 80.5kg or 12st 9½lbs. No question, I'm blowing up. Will I pull back later? Of course I will. No point in falling apart at this stage! But even when you're dieting you have to enjoy yourself now and then. If not frequently. Breakfast: bowl of berries, cappuccino with small amount of liquid sugar! Lunch by the pool: a Mentito, ham and melon – melons in Italy always taste

better than in London – and a vanilla and chocolate ice cream. Also one bread roll and half a breadstick. Dinner at Cip's Club restaurant, which is on a floating wooden platform in the grounds of the Cipriani. It looks out over the big canal to the main island on which most of Venice sits. I don't like the main dining room at the Cipriani much, but Cip's is terrific. There was a freebie starter of marinated sea bass. Then I had raw air-cured San Danieli ham with figs. Then roast fillet of sea bass with lemon and wild fennel. Very good Bellini, real peach juice. Finished with lemon sorbet. The Cipriani is on an island called Giudecca. The view is of Harry's Bar and the dreaded Hotel Monaco & Grand Canal as well as the church of Santa Maria della Salute, the Doge's Palace and the piazzetta that leads to St Mark's Square. Unique and great.

MONDAY 31 JULY

Morning weight 81.7kg or 12st 12lbs. What do you expect if you eat as I've been eating? Here's a two-and-a-half pound increase in one day! Breakfast: bowl of berries, cappuccino. Lunch at this marvellous table by the pool and overlooking the lagoon: home-made fusilli pasta with fresh tomato sauce, capers and mozzarella. Dessert of figs and a lemon sorbet, plus some biscuits. Dinner at Cip's. It's much better foo/*d than in the main Cipriani restaurant, where you're meant to wear a jacket even in the boiling heat of summer. I walked over to chat with David Frost there once and the restaurant manager said, 'You need a jacket.' I said, 'No one, not one man, is wearing a jacket.' 'They've got them hanging over the back of their chairs,' said the restaurant manager. What a nutcase! At Cip's you don't need a jacket. After the freebie starter of marinated sea bass I had San Danieli ham with figs. Then roast fillet of John Dory with lemon and wild fennel. A Bellini. Finished with a lemon pancake.

TUESDAY 1 AUGUST
Morning weight 81.7kg or 12st 12lbs. At least no increase! Breakfast: yoghurt with orange flower honey, cappuccino, half a croissant, a few bits of muesli without milk, strawberries and orange slices. All by the pool. Lunch: tagliolini with cheese and ham, a wild strawberry and raspberry tart. This was in the covered restaurant by the pool, as a great thunderstorm started about an hour before lunch. Luckily we had a tented pavilion. Two staff members with umbrellas rescued us and got us to the restaurant. After lunch the sun came out for the afternoon. We went to the cemetery where Diaghilev and various other notables are buried. It's on an island. Very atmospheric if you like tombstones, which I do. Back to Harry's Bar for dinner. Bellini. Cold sea bass with Russian salad. Fish risotto. Lemon sorbet. All superb.

WEDNESDAY 2 AUGUST
Morning weight 81.7kg or 12st 12lbs. Either the scales are stuck or my hour-long walks every evening are paying off. At least I'm not putting on any more weight. Breakfast by the pool: bowl of berries, yoghurt, cappuccino. Lunch: some breadsticks, mushroom omelette, Mentito cocktail, lemon sorbet and biscuits. Then took the private jet to London. Dinner: grilled sole, asparagus.

THURSDAY 3 AUGUST

Morning weight 80.3kg or 12st 9lbs. Not bad! Five pounds gained in six days in Venice eating like a pig. I'll get that off. Back to the old routine. Breakfast: 200g Woodlands organic live sheep's milk yoghurt, jam, clementine juice. 11-ish: coffee with crystal sugar, milk and single malt Scotch. Lunch: grilled sole, peas, carrots. Couple of bits of Rococo dairy-free and sugar-free chocolate around 5pm. Dinner, very exciting. Geraldine went to Peter Jones and bought a veggie juice-extractor machine. So we piled into it carrots, broccoli, ginger, cucumber, lettuce, apples and probably more, and out came – juice! I had some biscuity things with butter and some nuts and raisins. That was dinner! Then a walk in Holland Park. Then a lot of garden work. Night weight 79.3kg.

FRIDAY 4 AUGUST

Morning weight 79.7kg or 12st 7¾lbs. This is very odd! I have never known me to weigh more in the morning than in the evening before! But I weighed myself very carefully, and checked it more than once, both times! Anyway, it's in the right direction – down! Breakfast: 200g sheep's milk yoghurt, jam, clementine juice. 11-ish: coffee with single malt Scotch, milk and sugar. Lunch at The Wolseley, early, with Paola, who's up in town for her cancer checks. She is amazingly brave with what she's been through. She really is very ill. It makes you realise that if you have your health, shut up. Don't complain. Be grateful and get on with life. I had duck eggs on toast with mushrooms and bacon, a Buck's Fizz and summer pudding with clotted cream. Dinner: home-produced vegetable juice from my very own juicer, one apple added! Nuts and raisins. Bit of Rococo chocolate – separately, not bunged in the juicer. Night weight 80.5kg.

SATURDAY 5 AUGUST
Morning weight 79.1kg or 12st 6¼lbs. One and a half pounds off yesterday with summer pudding, clotted cream, bacon, toast etc.! 11-ish: coffee with single malt Scotch. Lunch at San Lorenzo, a very under-estimated place regarding food. Superb salami from Siena plus artichokes, then wild Scottish salmon with new potatoes, carrots and asparagus. No plate decoration, just simple and excellent. Unfortunately for my diet they have the best chocolate ice cream in the world. Mara, the boss, told me it had no preservatives so it only lasts two days. I had that plus some liquid lemon sorbet. Dinner: veggies juiced, plus nuts and raisins. Watched *Dirty Dancing*, the 1987 film in my cinema. Bloody good it is. Night weight 79.2kg. Bizarre! I only put on 0.1kg all day!

SUNDAY 6 AUGUST
Morning weight 77.7kg or 12st 3¼lbs. This weight is decreasing! Breakfast got very exciting – I added a bit of brown sugar to the sheep's milk yoghurt and jam, had orange juice and then, further, some raspberries with brown sugar! 11-ish: coffee with single malt Scotch, sugar, milk. To Michael Caine's for another perfect lunch. If only there were a restaurant serving food half as good! A Pimms, nuts, salmon – juicy and tasty, which it seldom ever is – cherry tomatoes, beans, some veg, fried, from Michael's garden, new potatoes. Then dessert of

two types of Häagen-Dazs ice cream, a cooked plum-type thing, and raspberries. Then biscuits but no tea. Back at home dug up bricks and tiles, laid them out and took damaged ones to the dump along with very heavy iron bars. Serious labour. Been doing it for a few days. Plus filling ex-log store with earth. Don't ask why. Dinner: veggie-extracted juice plus four chocolate biscuits. Night weight 79.2kg.

MONDAY 7 AUGUST
Morning weight 77.3kg or 12st 2½lbs. This is getting beyond ridiculous! I ate ice cream, lots of nuts at Michael Caine's, potatoes and other stuff, and here I am the next day not heavier at all! 11-ish: usual coffee with single malt Scotch. Lunch: grilled Dover sole, sweetcorn off the cob, beans. I added some butter. Around 4pm: iced coffee – no Scotch because I had a very important TV executive coming to discuss a TV show and I didn't want him to think I was a heavy drinker! Which, of course, I'm certainly not! Dinner: veggie-extracted juice, water biscuits buttered and with jam. Late, a banana! Night weight 79kg.

TUESDAY 8 AUGUST
Morning weight 77.4kg or 12st 2¾lbs. It's the late-eaten banana wot put on the extra quarter of a pound. I had my usual breakfast. 11-ish: coffee with single malt Scotch, milk, sugar. Lunch: grilled salmon, hollandaise sauce, peas and asparagus. Dinner: veggie-extracted juice. Water biscuits, jam and butter. Night weight 77.6kg.

WEDNESDAY 9 AUGUST

Morning weight 76.8kg or 12st 1¼lbs. I am disappearing! Another pound and a half down! All I can think of – if this is the area I stick in – I'm one stone (14 pounds to the forgetful) lower than my clothes are taken in for! It also proves the Fat Pig Diet really works! Breakfast: sheep's milk yoghurt with mixed berries (raspberries, blueberries and blackberries). As I'd not had my usual jam I had three teaspoonfuls of granulated brown sugar! Just like that! Lunch at The Wolseley. I threw caution to the winds! Complete bread roll with butter, Buck's Fizz, caviar omelette, a bit of Paola's scone with cream and jam, summer pudding with clotted cream. 5-ish: iced coffee with single malt Scotch, milk, white granulated sugar. Dinner: veggie juices extracted personally by me. It takes forever to get much liquid out of things like broccoli, lettuce and cabbage. Carrots are prolific juice-wise. I misjudged the whole thing anyway, produced far too much and ended up drinking two and half large glasses of the stuff plus water biscuits (rather a lot) with butter and jam. Night weight 78.6kg.

THURSDAY 10 AUGUST

Morning weight 78kg or 12st 4lbs. This is seriously odd! I ate a bit too much yesterday – but to go up two and three-quarter pounds in one day seems peculiar. Still, the scales don't lie. Or do they? Breakfast: the usual sheep's milk yoghurt, jam, clementine juice. 11-ish: the usual coffee with single malt Scotch and crystal sugar. Lunch: grilled sole, beans, carrots. In the afternoon I took 36 photos of myself on the automatic setting on my Leica, with the intention of one being used on the cover of my diet book. Dinner: veggie juice extracted by me, two crumpets with marmalade and butter! Very few nuts. I am being incautious. 11pm-ish: hot chocolate drink with brown granulated sugar. Night weight 78.1kg.

FRIDAY 11 AUGUST
Morning weight 77.2kg or 12st 2¼lbs. That's interesting, innit? Down one and three-quarter pounds on a day where I ate two crumpets for dinner covered in butter and marmalade and two hot drinks with sugar! But the bulk intake of the day was small. I think it proves my theory: eat less. Doesn't matter much what, just eat less. 11-ish: coffee with single malt Scotch, sugar, milk. Lunch: grilled lobster with lemon, some salad with Hellmann's mayonnaise. After lunch I drove the new Bentley Arnage, a £220,000 car, for *Five Drive*, a TV programme. A car's a car. But my Brioni blazer, which I put on for the event, and which was taken in very recently, now needs taking in again! Where will this all lead to? 4-ish: iced coffee with single malt Scotch, milk, white sugar. Dinner: one glass of veggie juice from juicer, water biscuits, butter, jam. Rather a lot! Before bed: hot chocolate drink with sugar. Night weight 80.2kg.

SATURDAY 12 AUGUST
Morning weight 77.2kg or 12st 2¼lbs. Hmmm. Please note this is down from 15 stone 10 pounds, which I used to be. A total weight loss of three stone seven and three-quarter pounds. Or 49.75 pounds. Or 22.6 kilograms. Just felt like bragging about it! Usual breakfast of sheep's

milk yoghurt, jam, clementine juice. 11-ish: coffee with sugar and single malt Scotch. Lunch at The Wolseley: fruit punch, chopped liver with water biscuits, butter and pickled cucumber, grilled plaice with potatoes and veggies, then Eton Mess, which is a rich creamy thing with meringue in it. The actress Una Stubbs was there. We've known each other for decades. She said she didn't recognise me because I'd lost so much weight. Dinner: veggie juice, nuts and raisins. Then I ate a crunchy bar that I'd found lurking among the staff food in the kitchen. And then another one! Then I watched an old movie, *The Bodyguard*, in my cinema. I'd missed it before. Bloody good. Night weight 80.2kg.

SUNDAY 13 AUGUST

Morning weight 77.2kg or 12st 2¼lbs. If I stay in this weight area I'm going to need my jackets and shirts taken in yet again. Slimming ain't cheap. Breakfast: orange juice (because I did it myself and I'm not sure where the clementines are kept; the oranges are in the fruit bowl!), sheep's milk yoghurt, jam, a handful of nuts and raisins. I picked Paola up from The Berkeley hotel, where the doorman stood and watched as she carried her case to my Suzuki Grand Vitara. He did nothing to help as she put the case in the back and got in. Pity. The hotel and its staff were doing very well until then. When I had taken her there in the Bentley last night the doorman was perfect. Obviously The Berkeley doormen are trained to ignore cheaper cars. On to the River Café, best food in London, for lunch: bruschetta, orange juice, linguine with figs, pigeon with veg, chocolate ice cream, white peach sorbet, limoncello, mint tea. A full lunch! Dinner: veggie juice, two pieces of buttered toast – one with peanut butter and banana, one just peanut butter. Then just before beddie-byes at about 11.30pm I did something really silly! I'd forgotten to take my Metformin and one other pill that you're meant to take with food. So I took a piece of brown bread, buttered it, added raspberry jam and had a jam sandwich! Then I went to bed. This is not high on the Fat Pig Diet for what you should do! Night weight 78.7kg.

MONDAY 14 AUGUST
Morning weight 77.6kg or 12st 3lbs. Up three-quarters of a pound. Bet the jam sandwich did it! Breakfast: the usual sheep's milk yoghurt, jam, clementine juice. 11-ish: the usual coffee with milk, brown crystal sugar and single malt Scotch. Lunch: grilled plaice, corn off the cob, peas. 4-ish: another coffee with Scotch. Dinner: plate of raw, fresh baby peas. My veggie juice drink. A few nuts. Then, again, a lapse! Around 9.30pm a jam sandwich with sliced banana on it! Naughty! Night weight 78.5kg.

TUESDAY 15 AUGUST
Morning weight 77.8kg or 12st 3½lbs. Up half a pound, and that's before Geraldine and I go to the South of France tomorrow, to a hotel with a two-Michelin-starred restaurant! I had my usual breakfast, then at 11-ish coffee with milk, sugar, single malt Scotch. Lunch: prawns with salad and Hellmann's mayonnaise. Coffee as usual

around 4pm. Dinner: veggie juice hand-crushed by my own hand on the cruncher, two pieces of buttered toast with jam and Philadelphia cream cheese. Before bed hot chocolate with milk and sugar. Night weight 78.5kg.

WEDNESDAY 16 AUGUST
Morning weight 77.8kg or 12st 3½lbs. The next 19 days will be a real test of my willpower. We're going to La Réserve de Beaulieu, a great hotel in the unspoilt coastal town of Beaulieu, east of Nice, which adjoins another totally unspoilt little place called St Jean Cap Ferrat. They are as the South of France used to be – as opposed to most of the rest, which is overbuilt beyond belief. La Réserve's restaurant has two Michelin stars. Veggie juice dinners will not be available. If I can come back only 10 pounds up on what I am now it'll be a miracle. That would still leave me in my comfort weight zone. Usual breakfast. Lunch at home: fish and two green veg. Then on the private jet I had two packets of crisps! Dinner at La Réserve de Beaulieu, one of the best hotels in the world: crayfish appetiser, melon, rabbit from Brest stuffed with apricots and fresh almonds served with a little pastry, young carrots and candied white onions, then a pre-dessert of fruit and crème de cacao mousse and four tiny ice creams in cones, then a lemon sorbet and some toffee petits fours. Not a slimming meal. Night weight 77.5kg on the hotel scales.

THURSDAY 17 AUGUST
Morning weight 77.5kg or 12st 2¾lbs. This weight I rather doubt. I think the hotel scales are more flattering

than mine at home. But as they're all I've got, I'll diligently record what they say! Breakfast overlooking the sparkling sea: piece of white baguette, croissant, orange juice, coffee. The baguette was rubbery. I told them in no uncertain terms this was not a two-Michelin-star baguette; it was a railway station baguette. They assured me it wouldn't happen again. Very hot sun all day. Lunch by the pool and overlooking the sea. On the left the high cliffs, on the right the lovely gardens, villas and distant port of St Jean Cap Ferrat, and David Niven's pink villa now re-sold to someone else. Nothing modern or unpleasant in the view. I ate a salade niçoise, bit of roll and butter, mint sorbet. Dinner: foie gras with fruits of the season, courgettes with king prawns, a freebie starter of shellfish with a veggie soup poured over it. No dessert. Just three toffees. A baby was let in in a high chair and started screaming. I fled. Didn't take night weight!

FRIDAY 18 AUGUST

Morning weight 77.6kg or 12st 3lbs. Very hot again. Breakfast of croissant and coffee by the pool. Lunch by the pool: vegetable omelette, beautifully done, with creamed spinach on the side and grilled tomatoes. A mini baguette with olive oil. Petits fours. Dinner: turbot and langoustines from Brittany roasted with almonds, home-made tomato sauce, ginger and marjoram. Pre-dessert, the little ice cream cones again, a peach granita and a little madeleine cake. Main dessert, a lemon soufflé. Then four wrapped toffees from the petits fours trolley. Will this be the end of the diet, and me? Didn't dare take night weight.

SATURDAY 19 AUGUST

Very difficult to see the weight on the hotel scales. They've got this silly needle thing that points, not electric numbers like at home. Geraldine checked it. 78kg or 12st 4lbs. Going up, as I expected! Breakfast: part of a baguette with butter and jam, a sort of chocolate cup cake, sheep's milk yoghurt and jam, orange juice, coffee. Mid-morning: a lemon pressé with white sugar galore. Lunch: salade niçoise, bit of baguette with olive oil, dessert of wild strawberries and a mint sorbet. Another citron pressé with sugar in the afternoon. Dinner: shrimps and loup de mer (this is sea bass, I think) with veggies. Before that some tiny starter things, a Buck's Fizz, freebie starter of frog's legs with a garlic mousse. Dessert was wild strawberries, raspberries and mint sorbet, then a few petits fours.

SUNDAY 20 AUGUST

Morning weight 78.5kg or 12st 5lbs. Inevitably blowing up! Breakfast: sheep's milk yoghurt with jam, bit of baguette, coffee, orange juice. Later, two citron pressés with sugar as I waited for our lunch guest, Andrew Neil, who was stuck in a traffic jam at Villefranche. It's a narrow coastal road and there's a traffic light as you enter Villefranche, which produces a terrible tailback. I once drove on the wrong side of the road, past all the cars, over the red light and straight into the arms of six French policemen waiting in a small garden area! I always carry a little brochure used at film festivals, showing me with my director's chair and with a mini biography in three languages. The police read this and kept asking questions about Charles Bronson, and I had a photo taken with the leading detective. They wished me well as I drove off. Very nice of them. But I never did that again! Lunch: melon and ham (the melons are superb – much better than any I've ever had in London). Then goujons of turbot and a little bread. I told Andrew I had started dieting in Barbados when my tooth cap came loose and cut into my tongue so it pained me to eat. He said, 'Could you speak?' I said, 'Yes.' He said, 'That's a pity. We could have had two for the price of one!' Witty lad, Andrew. Dinner: melon and ham, a Buck's Fizz, some bread, pre-dessert of pineapple jelly and fruit cocktail with a mousse of pina colada and these little ice cream cones (I had them every dinner at La Réserve). Mint sorbet and wild strawberries as main dessert. Then three chocolate-coated slices of orange peel.

MONDAY 21 AUGUST

Morning weight 79kg or 12st 6lbs. 'Going up!' as they say in lifts. Or used to! Breakfast: one half little pain aux raisin (that's bread with raisins), coffee, orange juice. I told them I thought their orange juice came out of a plastic carton. They denied it. I said I wanted it freshly squeezed by hand seconds before it was served to me. Thereafter it tasted quite different! I also had sheep's milk yoghurt with jam. The previous day the assistant restaurant manager had just plonked a supermarket yoghurt on the table. I only had one plate with crumbs on it. I gave him my views very clearly. This morning I had a plate as well as a bowl for the yoghurt and extra spoons. Lunch: tagliatelli with an enormous piece of mozzarella on top (odd that!) and tomato. Bread with olive oil. John Gold, my guest, ordered salade niçoise but got a Caesar salad from the same twit who gave me yoghurt with no bowl to eat it from at breakfast. Then mint sorbet with wild strawberries, blueberries and raspberries. Petits fours also, which came too late. At La Réserve (as well as at some other French hotels) there is no dinner served – other than room service – on a Monday night! This in high season! It's because of the 35-hour working week, which is making life impossible for French hoteliers. So Geraldine and I were cast out into the street for our dinner. We walked up the main street of Beaulieu, a very nice spot, the Boulevard Maréchal Leclerc. Didn't want anything grand. We ended up in Le Berlugan 'cuisine traditionelle' grill bar brasserie. The speciality of the day was English fillet of cod and chips. I had a small part of an enormous pizza ardechoise with tomatoes, raw ham and lots of other stuff. It was very good but the place was alive with screaming kids. A nightmare. I had a fruit cocktail, which tasted like all tinned fruit juices bunged together. That was it. Quite enough.

TUESDAY 22 AUGUST

Morning weight 78.5kg or 12st 5lbs. See, had hardly any dinner and lost weight. Be aware! Breakfast: proper orange juice (because I'd complained before), various bits of bread and stuff. Different sheep's milk yoghurt, not as good. Jam. Coffee. A lemon pressé mid-morning with white sugar. Lunch: roll with olive oil, salade niçoise, wild strawberries and mint sorbet. I am a creature of habit. Dinner with Sir Roger Moore, his wife Kristina, son

Geoffrey and his wife at the Hotel Metropole in Monte Carlo – Restaurant Joël Robuchon. One of Joël's chain of restaurants, this is largely run by the chef who used to be at La Réserve (he was good, but not nearly as good as Olivier, who followed him). I ordered a strawberry Bellini and the waiter said, snootily, 'It's a Rossini!' The special that night was roasted baby goat. I love goat. Only had it once, on the beach in Jamaica in 1974. Been waiting to find it on a menu ever since. It was terrific here too. I had it with mashed potato. To start I had melon and some of Geraldine's very good smoked salmon. The wait for the main course goat was ridiculously long. Ended up with a Grand Marnier soufflé with ice cream. It was excellent.

WEDNESDAY 23 AUGUST

Morning weight 78.5kg or 12st 5lbs. Interesting. Here I am eating piggishly and I'm still only 12 stone five pounds. Either the hotel scales are wrong or I'm I don't know what. We'll see for sure when I get back to my London scales. Breakfast: goat's milk yoghurt, jam, wild strawberries, blueberries, raspberries, some bread, a sort of pastry thing with apple in it, coffee, orange juice. Lunch by the pool: Parma ham and a large melon, mint sorbet with mixed berries. Spoke to Julian Lennon, who was visiting. Hadn't seen him since he stayed at Sandy Lane, Barbados, a few years ago. Dinner at La Hostellerie Jérôme in La Turbie with Gerald and Rachel de Thame. He's a seriously big commercial director; she was a top model who now does gardening columns and TV appearances as a gardening expert. Hostellerie Jérôme is a marvellous, two-Michelin-star restaurant high in the hills above Cap d'Ail. I started with canapés and a Buck's Fizz. Then artichoke salad. Then langoustines roasted with foie gras and potiron, which is a kind of small pumpkin with a chestnut taste. Before that a freebie starter of duck in pastry served with rocket sauce and salad. Dessert was a millefeuille of wild strawberries. Then we got a freebie lemon sorbet and some petits fours. This is a sensational restaurant!

THURSDAY 24 AUGUST

Morning weight 77.6kg or 12st 3lbs. Work that out! Can it possibly be right or are the hotel scales favouring thinnie-Winnie rather strongly? I mean, how can I eat what I ate yesterday and lose weight? Breakfast: small piece of chocolate cake, goat's milk yoghurt with jam, bit of bread roll, orange juice, coffee. Lunch by the pool: salade niçoise with melon on the side. I wouldn't let them put the bread basket on the table because if they did I'd eat some. Dessert of berries (no sugar), mint sorbet. Later I had a lemon pressé with white sugar. Dinner at the house of Leslie Bricusse, a friend I've known since Cambridge, who wrote 'What Kind of Fool Am I?' and other hits, has three Oscars and is a great chef. Other guests at his villa in St Paul de Vence were Michael Caine, Roger Moore and Bill Wyman. I had a few nuts, a bit of white wine, barbecued shrimps with a very good sauce, lamb Moroccan style with salad, tomatoes and grilled figs, apple tart and cream. Only trouble with dining with Leslie is he's in a gated estate and although he gives you a password it never works and I'm always trapped. I couldn't make the password numbers work on the dark panel by the gate. Then Sir Frank Lowe, a top advertising man, and his lady friend Pat Booth, a novelist, came along from the dinner. 'Frank'll get us out,' said Geraldine, as if I was incompetent. He tried and failed. 'Roger Moore got out,' observed Pat Booth. 'He's James Bond for heaven sake. He leapt over the gate!' said Frank testily. In the end I had to go back to the house to get Leslie to come and open it with his remote control device!

FRIDAY 25 AUGUST
Morning weight still 77.6kg or 12st 3lbs. I still find this hard to believe! Breakfast: a baguette with butter and jam, a 'chocolate bread' called pain au chocolat, bit of watermelon, sheep's milk yoghurt with jam, coffee, orange juice. Lunch at the hotel with impresario Adam Kenwright and his girlfriend Katherine: salade niçoise, mixed berries and mint sorbet, a couple of petits fours. Later a citron pressé with white sugar. Dinner with Adam and Katherine and Geraldine. Geraldine and I had started on the terrace of La Réserve, which is so beautiful and overlooks the bay and the sea. But it was a bit windy! In fact it was close to a howling gale. So the staff moved everyone inside to the elegant dining room. About 20 minutes later the wind subsided but we were in by then! I had lobster salad and a breast of chicken, all fairly fancily done as it's a two-Michelin-star restaurant. I also had a little bread and a lemon soufflé.

SATURDAY 26 AUGUST
Morning weight 77.6kg or 12st 3lbs. Still don't believe it! Breakfast: berries, bit of baguette, orange juice, coffee.

Lunch by the pool: salade niçoise with melon, bit of bread with olive oil, petits fours. Dinner at La Chaumière, one of my all-time favourite restaurants. It's high on the Grande Corniche. Very farmhouse style. A set menu that is always superbly done. Ham, melon, tomatoes, aubergine pâté, boiled eggs, crudités (which are raw vegetables) with a wonderful creamy sauce. Rough meat pâté. Slices of the best beef ever with jacket potato and butter. Incredible strawberry jelly with clotted cream you take with a ladle from an enormous bucket. A citron pressé with white sugar. How can my weight be the same after this?

SUNDAY 27 AUGUST
Morning weight 78.2kg or 12st 4½lbs. The scales do move then! I increased! Breakfast: berries, some baguette with butter and jam, coffee, orange juice. Lunch by the pool: vegetable omelette, bit of baguette with butter, mint sorbet. Dinner with Adam and Katherine back at La Hostellerie Jérôme: onion and tomato tart, a little freebie pie of duck with summer truffle sauce and green veg. Main course, pigeon de Lauragais, which is, apparently, a place near Toulouse. That's where the pigeon came from! Whether it flew or came by train, I don't know. Then I had a lemon and a mascarpone sorbet. Then an ice cream and some petits fours that were incredible.

MONDAY 28 AUGUST
Morning weight 78.2kg or 12st 4½lbs. I still find these scales generous, to say the least. Breakfast: I had rather too many pieces of bread and rolls. Also goat's milk

yoghurt with jam, orange juice, coffee. Lunch: cold soup called gazpacho, a whole melon and a mint sorbet plus petits fours. Dinner back at La Chaumière with Elton John, David Furnish and Michael and Shakira Caine. Elton and I go way back. I made the first record of his that was ever released. It was for my 1969 Olympic epic *The Games*. Stanley Baker and Mona Washbourne were in a house in Windsor and Stanley was persuading Michael Crawford (playing a milkman) to enter for the Olympic marathon. We had a background voice coming out of a radio. The song on the radio, *From Denver to LA*, was by Francis Lai, who composed the music for *Love Story* and *A Man and a Woman*. We had a session singer record it. But when I saw the film I thought the voice was grating, so I asked for it to be re-done with another singer. My music booker, David Katz, rang me one evening from CTS Studios, then in Bayswater, and reported, 'I've got Reg Dwight here. He has a very melodious voice. Do you want to hear him before we record him? He's prepared to audition.' I said, 'Just get on with it.' Reg Dwight was, of course, Elton John before he changed his name. He was terrific. Then Elton had an album come out and became famous. When *The Games* was released 20th Century Fox put out the album, with *From Denver to LA* credited to 'singer Elton Johns', mis-spelt with an s. Elton's record company sued Fox saying, 'You didn't employ Elton John, you employed Reg Dwight. Withdraw the record.' So 20th Century Fox did. About 15 years ago I bought a copy on the New York black market for £600 and presented it to Elton. He remembered not only the recording but the exact fee he got! Back to my food!

Don't forget it's a set menu, so it was the pâté, the crudités and vegetable salad, but this time I had lamb chop (you can choose between beef and lamb and if you order in advance they'll get a chicken). It's all roasted on the open fire in front of you. Then I had the strawberry jelly again plus a little bit of their fantastic apple pie and cream.

TUESDAY 29 AUGUST
Morning weight 78kg or 12st 4lbs. I wish I had these scales at home. I'm sure they're kind to me! Breakfast: part of a baguette, some other bread stuff, goat's milk yoghurt, jam, orange juice, coffee. We were visited by the wonderfully unusual Fausto Allegri, Guest Relations manager of the Hotel Splendido in Portofino. He came to lunch. Fausto's long-running gag when I go to Portofino is to say, 'La Réserve has closed down!' He likes his little joke, does Fausto. For lunch I was very good. I had salade niçoise, bread and olive oil, a mint sorbet. Dinner was with the wonderful singer and guitarist Chris Rea, his wife Joan and daughter Julia. Probably the brightest teenager I've ever met. He chose Pulcinella in Monte Carlo. Monte Carlo to me is like a council estate. Endless high-rise flats. Nothing like the elegant, villa-strewn place I used to know. Pulcinella is under an underpass, or almost. I had been there before. Rod Stewart was there that time. Apparently, according to Chris, it's much used by the motor racing fraternity. Chris loves fast cars. Once had 11 Ferraris. We had a pizza freebie starter. Then I had tagliolini du chef, which was fresh noodles with ham, tomato, mushrooms and cream. Then a veal

escalope with lemon, chips and lettuce. Chris took my chips as I couldn't eat them on my diet, although I tried two. I had a honey and cream cake with walnuts on top, which Chris said was called a dartboard. Not sure I believe him. Also a tiny bit of tiramisu. Not a madly slimming dinner. And being dinner it was less slimming than ever.

WEDNESDAY 30 AUGUST
Morning weight 79kg or 12st 6lbs. I am, like the sun, rising. Weight is increasing. No surprise! Two pounds up in one day! Breakfast: quite a bit of bread, sheep's milk yoghurt with jam, orange juice, coffee. Lunch: tomato omelette, grilled tomato, two sausages, mixed berries, mint sorbet. Ben Frow, a total delight, who is in charge of features and documentaries for Channel 5, arrived. We discussed my proposed TV series. For dinner he came with us and Chris, Joan and Julia Rea to La Chaumière. Horror of horrors! I'd forgotten my credit cards. So Ben started our holiday together by paying for six people! Disgraceful of me! Set menu don't forget, so I had Parma ham and melon, raw veggies, pâté (one of meat, one of aubergine), leg of lamb, baked potato, butter, strawberry jelly and cream. Very nice meal. Great company.

THURSDAY 31 AUGUST
Morning weight 79kg or 12st 6lbs. Breakfast: croissant, orange juice, butter, jam. Lunch by the pool of salade niçoise and lemon sorbet. Dinner at La Hostellerie Jérôme. Again. But it's so good! I had foie gras with figs, médaillon de veau with artichokes and olive oil and a lot

of other stuff. The duck pie for freebie starter. Then lemon and mascarpone sorbets and coffee ice cream and petit fours. This time I had my credit card and paid!

FRIDAY 1 SEPTEMBER

Morning weight 79kg or 12st 6lbs. Bizarre. I should be getting heavier! Breakfast: usual baguette with jam and butter, pain au chocolat, tiny bit of coffee, orange juice, sheep's milk yoghurt and jam. Lunch at La Colombe d'Or in St Paul de Vence. One of the greatest places on earth. This is where then-impoverished artists – Picasso, Braque and others – paid by leaving paintings. The oils on display in the rustic dining room are probably worth £50 million at least. In summer you lunch on the terrace. It's on the edge of the medieval village of St Paul de Vence. I remember it when people lived in all the buildings. Now most of the ground floors are shops, selling quite classy tat. The whole place is still enchanting. We took Ben Frow. We all had their famous hors d'oeuvre, which comes in so many little bowls it's impossible to count them – sausages, herrings, rice with raisins, everything you could want and more. The loup de mer, which is sea bass, tastes better here than anywhere, with a rich yellow sauce and boiled potatoes. Then a striped ice cream that is sometimes called cassata (they give it a fancy name). Dinner was with Ben Frow at La Réserve de Beaulieu. I had a freebie starter of shrimp. Then melon, roast duck, a lemon soufflé with lemon sorbet.

SATURDAY 2 SEPTEMBER

Morning weight 79kg or 12st 6lbs. Breakfast: baguette with jam and butter, little chocolate cake, sheep's milk yoghurt with jam, orange juice, coffee. Lunch by pool: goat's cheese salad with melon and ham on the side. Dessert, mint sorbet, mixed berries and some petits fours. Dinner on retail genius tycoon Sir Philip Green's yacht, beautifully decorated by his wife Tina. This has a crew of 22. It was parked near the coast of St Jean Cap Ferrat, very near our hotel. I had Buck's Fizz, crab cakes, skewered beef and chicken satay, then lamb cutlets with green veggies, cauliflower cheese and mashed potatoes, and finished with a superb bread and butter pudding. The last time I had a meal with Philip Green personally (other than at events) was fish and chips in bhs in Oxford Street. They were very good, too.

SUNDAY 3 SEPTEMBER

Morning weight 79kg or 12st 6lbs. Breakfast: part of a baguette with jam and butter, part of a pain au chocolat, sheep's milk yoghurt with jam, coffee, orange juice, two kumquats. In fact I've been eating a lot of kumquats in the room for days! Sir Frank Lowe, an exceptionally nice person and advertising agency genius, and his lady friend Pat Booth joined us for lunch by the pool of La Réserve. I had salade niçoise, tiny bit of bread, melon and a coupe chocolate, which was ice cream with cream and chocolate sauce and other things around it. And a limoncello aperitif. For dinner I had tomato soup, turbot with king prawns and a vanilla soufflé.

MONDAY 4 SEPTEMBER

Morning weight 79kg or 12st 6lbs. I do not believe this! It's my last morning weigh-in on the Réserve de Beaulieu hotel scales. Tomorrow the awful truth will out when I return to my own scales at home. Breakfast: bit of baguette, sheep's milk yoghurt and jam, some other bread stuff, coffee, orange juice. After 19 days of sunshine I was almost glad to see it cloudy on the drive to Nice airport. 'Missed that!' I thought. Private jet left Nice 20 minutes late because they were waiting to be given fuel. A nice young man from England, working for the firm that meets, greets and sees people off, told me this was normal at Nice. It's never happened to me before. We had to land at Farnborough because the runway at RAF Northolt (half an hour nearer my house) was being re-surfaced or something. On the plane I ate one medium-sized pack of Walker's salted crisps. Getting into my 1966 Rolls Royce Phantom V, which was waiting by the steps of the private jet (it's the sort of car the Queen is driven around in), I noticed it was rusting like mad under the doors. Major fortune coming to tart it up! You think the rich have it easy? Forget it! Lunch at home: grilled salmon, runner beans. 4-ish: coffee with single malt Scotch, sugar, milk. Dinner: back on the old routine – large glass of freshly extracted veggie juice (I added a bit of double cream), some fresh organic raw peas. Night weight 80.5kg. This means I've no chance whatsoever of being the 12 stone six pounds I've miraculously and diligently – and inaccurately – been recording for the last few days.

TUESDAY 5 SEPTEMBER

Morning weight 79.5kg or 12st 7½lbs. Not as bad as I feared. Did I put on one and a quarter pounds yesterday? Or were the hotel scales in France pretty accurate after all? I think a one-and-a-half-pound increase is unlikely. Either way, I need to lose. I've decided my new weight will be – wait for it! – not in the previous comfort zone of 12 stone 12 pounds to 13 stone two pounds, BUT hovering around 12 stone three pounds! This is a totally new aim. A major escalation of dieting. All my jackets will have to be taken in yet again! Breakfast: sheep's milk yoghurt, jam and clementine juice. 11-ish: coffee and Scotch. Lunch: grilled sole, corn off the cob with butter, beans. Checked the draft cover for this book, which was later changed when the publisher changed. A leading bookshop didn't like the face-photo I took of myself on the automatic camera setting (adapted into a pig!). 4pm-ish: the coffee and Scotch routine. Dinner: veggie-extracted juice with cream added, water biscuits with butter and jam, fresh raw peas. Went for a one-hour walk in Holland Park. Night weight 80.3kg.

WEDNESDAY 6 SEPTEMBER

Morning weight 79.1kg or 12st 6¼lbs. Coming down. But I've lowered the bar. Having decided to be on or around 12 stone three pounds – and that being on the cover of this book – I could be in the poo! I have to keep weight down to that area. Will readers rush up to me in the street, rip my clothes off (still not a pretty sight!) and dump me on a scales to see if I really am 12 stone three pounds? Will they demand a refund in cash for their book if I am not? Will I stand the mental strain of it all? Watch this space – where nothing will happen. Just wait and see! Breakfast: sheep's milk yoghurt, jam, clementine juice. 11-ish: coffee, single malt Scotch. Lunch: lamb cutlets, one roast potato, veggies. 4-ish: coffee with single malt Scotch. Dinner: veggie juice, six chocolate biscuits; later one slice of bread and jam. Night weight 79.6kg.

THURSDAY 7 SEPTEMBER
Morning weight 79kg or 12st 6lbs. A tiny decrease. Breakfast: goat's milk yoghurt, jam, clementine juice. 11-ish: coffee with single malt Scotch. Lunch: grilled sole, two green veggies. 4pm-ish: coffee with single malt Scotch. Tonight I have to eat out at Cipriani with Peter Wood, the brilliant boss of esure, to discuss a possible (I say no more than possible) return of my 'Calm Down Dear' commercials. The computerised mouse that took over from me was not a success. Sales plummeted. Then they tried another type of ad, which I thought very dull. Peter suggested I might join that ad as a kind of interviewer. To sort of spruce it up. He's writing a script and I'll consider it. I was utterly stupid at this dinner. I ate far too much. I started with tagliolini with ham and cheese, then a Dover sole and then a thin slice of cream pie. Finished with mint tea, at least no sugar. A ridiculous meal. I'm meant to be on a diet! Night weight 79.5kg.

FRIDAY 8 SEPTEMBER
Morning weight 78.8kg or 12st 5¾lbs. Breakfast: goat's milk yoghurt, jam, clementine juice. 11-ish: coffee with single malt Scotch. Lunch: grilled sole, two green

veggies. 4pm-ish: coffee with single malt Scotch. Dinner: tired of juicing veggies I went mad and cut up lots of raw veggies to have as a salad. Added olive oil and then, foolishly, Brie cheese and Parmesan cheese. Night weight 79.5kg.

SATURDAY 9 SEPTEMBER

Morning weight 78.8kg or 12st 5¾lbs. Breakfast: sheep's milk yoghurt, jam, clementine juice. Lunch at The Wolseley: one bread roll and butter, smoked salmon, lamb shank with mashed potatoes, apple and rhubarb crumble with cream, small espresso. Not exactly a dieter-lunch. Dinner: veggie-extracted juice. One small bag of roast salted nuts. Before bed: one iced chocolate drink with sugar. Checked through some more of my clothes, having given seven jackets to the alterations tailor on Friday. It's unbelievable! Jackets taken in in July are now much too big! Even the sleeves are having to be taken in because when the jacket was made I was fatter all round! I have to keep around 12 stone three pounds to 12 stone six pounds now or I'm dead clotheswise. In the evening I cut up some logs with an electric saw. Miracle I didn't cut my leg off. Night weight 79.5kg.

SUNDAY 10 SEPTEMBER

Morning weight 78.8kg or 12st 5¾lbs. Breakfast: Coco-Pops cereal, sugar, milk, clementine juice. I thought it a bit odd, on reading the *Sunday Times*, to see they list all their prominent writers in an ad with little photos of them. I am excluded! Yet I've been writing for them for longer than anyone else (since 1970) and my column is regularly shown to be the second most read in MORI polls, year after year. Are they trying to tell me something? Lunch at Michael Caine's house in Surrey. Always a terrible, but super-tasty, temptation. A Pimms and unsalted nuts. Grilled salmon, marvellous new potatoes from his garden, some green veg I'm not clever enough to identify, something called a Hello Dolly made by his daughter Natasha (sort of cakey it is), figs in cream with peaches, tiny bit of ice cream, some after-dinner mint choccies. Then I had a problem for a man on a diet – dinner at The Wolseley with Christian and Christine Roberts. Christian owns my favourite restaurant in Barbados. He had been disturbed to see a junior partner and minority shareholder, a man named Steve Cox, with whom he has been in litigation for three years, describing himself on the internet as 'Managing Director and owner of the Lone Star restaurant in Barbados'. Christian owns it in that he's the majority shareholder (over 50 per cent) and he said Steve was not the Managing Director either. Oh well, partnerships, whether equal or not, often go wrong. No one ever plans for a dispute when they set up together. It's all going to be rosy. They'll be friends forever. This seldom happens, but there is usually no exit strategy on paper, so it ends in friction, litigation and disaster. I've seen it again and again. My dinner was a bit of a disaster. I had a bit of a bread roll with butter, 80 grams of Beluga caviar with a blini, sour cream and a small bit of toast, and an excellent vanilla milkshake. Not as slimming as my normal veggie juice. But it could have been worse. Night weight 80kg.

MONDAY 11 SEPTEMBER

Morning weight 78.8kg or 12st 5¾lbs. Hanging in. I'd like to be two and half pounds lighter! Breakfast: sheep's milk yoghurt, jam, clementine juice. 11-ish: coffee with single malt Scotch. Lunch: grilled sole, corn on the cob taken off the cob with large pat of butter, tomato sauce, beans. 4pm-ish: Scotch with coffee mixed with drinking chocolate. Dinner: vegetable juice, nuts. Night weight 79.9kg.

TUESDAY 12 SEPTEMBER

Morning weight 78.7kg or 12st 5½lbs. Breakfast: coffee-Scotch-chocolate. Then total fiasco! Left house at 6.45am to go to Battersea heliport to get helicopter to Manchester for one of my police ceremonies, this one to have a memorial unveiled by his widow for DC Stephen Oake, who was stabbed to death by a terrorist. At 7.30am the heliport had a phone call from the helicopter pilot, from a firm called Aeromega, that he was stranded in Sussex and couldn't take off because of cloud. Yet the previous evening I'd agreed an extra £1,000 to upgrade the helicopter to one that could fly in cloud! As there was also trouble in Manchester with the weather, I decided to drive. The ceremony was at 11am. Then I was told it could take four hours (particularly at rush hour and in a 1966 Rolls Phantom!) so I tried to get a jet plane. Couldn't find one. Tried for a propeller plane from Oxford. But that airport was closed because of mist. So for the first time in my 33 ceremonies I didn't get there. The Deputy Chief Constable of Manchester read my speech! When I later remonstrated with Howard Mersey of Aeromega, asking why, if there was a likely problem, they didn't call me at home at 6am so I could re-arrange things, he said, 'We didn't have your number.' 'You phoned me three times yesterday and twice the day before!' I exploded. 'We forgot to give it to the operations room' was his lame excuse. In future, rather than use Aeromega, I'll hitchhike! So I've arranged to go up by jet (which turned out to be cheaper than the helicopter!) on Saturday to lay flowers at the memorial with DC Oake's widow and children. I'll have lunch in Manchester. That'll be interesting! Lunch today: grilled salmon, fresh peas, asparagus. 4-ish: usual coffee-chocolate-Scotch. Dinner: small glass of vegetable juice, salted nuts. Then went to an art exhibition of paintings by talented Adam Bricusse, son of Leslie, who wrote many enormous hits including 'Candy Man' and 'Talk to the Animals'. Then had a glass of red wine and some unsalted nuts and raisins on my balcony at home. Pretty desperate for a Marmite sandwich at 11pm but Geraldine stopped me having it! Night weight 79.3kg.

WEDNESDAY 13 SEPTEMBER
Morning weight 78.3kg or 12st 4½lbs. Bit of abstemious-ness pays off. Dropped a pound! Breakfast: sheep's milk yoghurt, jam, clementine juice. 11-ish: coffee-chocolate-Scotch. Lunch: crabmeat and salad. 5-ish Scotch-coffee-choccie mix. Dinner at the River Café with Michael and Shakira Caine. This is highly dangerous. I don't usually go out on Wednesday! Started with a strawberry Bellini, then fig salad with some green leaves, then ravioli stuffed with some sort of meat, then a white peach sorbet. 'Why

is the white peach sorbet pink?' asked Michael Caine. Why indeed! I finished with a limoncello liqueur. The River Café is undoubtedly the best food in London. Afterwards Lady Ruth Rogers, co-owner and sometime chef at the River Café (she was cooking that night), took us to hubby Lord Rogers' architect offices adjacent for a look around. Night weight 79.3kg.

THURSDAY 14 SEPTEMBER

Morning weight 78.3kg or 12st 4½lbs. Surprised I didn't put on something having gone out to dinner. Breakfast: usual sheep's milk yoghurt, jam, clementine juice. 11-ish: choccie-coffee-Scotch. Had an article in the *Spectator* today, which I, with no modesty, thought was very funny. It was about my brushes with the taxman, including when I did something very naughty in the late 1960s when tax was 98p in the pound. Years later I told the Revenue and happily paid them three million pounds in unpaid tax and interest! The *Daily Mail* asked me to re-do the article for them but I said 'No thanks'. The *Evening Standard* quoted it widely. I have a feeling others will too. It involves the bizarre contention by a revenue inspector in Tyne and Wear that my lunches and dinners for articles in the *Sunday Times* are not deductible because I also eat to live and therefore there is duality of purpose. So meals could not be deducted as a legitimate business expense. Got a quarter of my £5,000 investment in Andrew Lloyd Webber's production of *Evita* back. That's unusual. Mostly I lose all monies I put into theatre. This time I only lost most of it! Lunch: chilli con carne with all the trimmings. 5-ish: Scotch-coffee-choccie. Dinner: only freshly extracted veggie juice drink, one glassful! Then succumbed just before going to bed and had a Marmite sandwich with butter – one piece of brown bread doubled over! Night weight 79.1kg.

FRIDAY 15 SEPTEMBER

Morning weight: 77.9kg or 12st 3¾lbs. That was at 6.45am. I weighed myself three times to be sure. Then I did three-quarters of an hour gardening, into the jacuzzi and the swimming pool, came back to the scales (having eaten absolutely nothing) and now weighed 78.2kg! This often happens, I notice. Your very first weight on waking up rises, even though you eat no more. About 45 minutes later, after breakfast of 200g of sheep's milk yoghurt, jam and clementine juice, my weight had risen to 78.6kg! 11-ish: usual coffee-Scotch-chocolate. Lunch at The Wolseley. I had a whole roll-stick thing with butter, a fillet streak with two new potatoes, an apple crumble with cream, and a tiny bit of Princess's Sachertorte. There was a court case in Vienna over Sachertorte, which was made at the Hotel Sacher. They stopped the name being used on stuff not made there, but there was some loophole. So perhaps The Wolseley won't be sued! Lady Rogers of the River Café was eating there too. I had a big lunch, but veggie-juice dinner'll deal with it. Dinner: veggie juice and, just before bed, a Marmite sandwich! Night weight 80kg.

SATURDAY 16 SEPTEMBER

Morning weight 78.3kg or 12st 4½lbs. Breakfast: one piece of bread with marmalade, coffee-Scotch-chocolate-milk-sugar. Off early for private jet to Manchester to put flowers at the memorial for DC Stephen Oake in Crumpsall Lane. (Aeromega helicopters have now sent a grovelling letter of apology for letting me down. Means nothing to me.) In the lounge at Farnborough airport had a bag of crisps! I was met in Manchester by marvellous second-hand Rolls and Bentley dealer, Steve Gallimore, in an immaculate 1996 Brooklands Bentley. He'd just sold it for £26,000! Very good value. After laying my flowers and talking to local police and the press and TV, I went off to lunch in Rochdale. Not many people take a private jet to and from lunch in Rochdale. Makes life interesting. The place was called Nutters. The chef is Andrew Nutter. His dad Rodney, bow-tied and in evening dress, serves and runs the room with ma Jean. There was me, Geraldine, local policeman, Inspector Julian Snowball, and his wife Sheila (Julian had very efficiently run the ceremony with us) and Steve our car dealer. It's a nice old 1860 house set in big grounds. Starter was the best pieces of Welsh rarebit I've ever had, plus some smoked salmon canapés – but big ones – plus a plate of bits and pieces. I then had scallops with black pudding and olive oil-mashed potatoes. Very, very pleasant. The slivers of black pudding from Bury were a bit too slivery. Couldn't taste them much. To finish I had poached plums with crumble on top and an ice cream. Good meal. Back at home a long walk in the park, then just veggie juice plus some water biscuits, jam and butter. Bit of night-time gardening. Then before bed a coconut Actimel drink and some strawberries without cream or sugar. Night weight 79kg.

SUNDAY 17 SEPTEMBER

Morning weight 78.3kg or 12st 4½lbs. Can't seem to get below that for the moment. Breakfast: orange juice (yes orange, not clementine! I do it myself on Sunday!), sheep's milk yoghurt, jam. This is the first morning of the re-designed back page of the *Sunday Times* News Review. They've cut editorial things down to make room for an advert! Bloody cheek! My column is the same number of words but the photo is much smaller. Even sadder by far is that they've more than halved the number of words available for readers' letters. I think they're the best thing in the paper. I shall ask the editor to give them more room. Worth a try! I considered throwing myself from the basement window. It was a close call, but I decided against it. Lunch at Michael Caine's. There were some traffic jams on the drive down to his residence looking over the Surrey hills. I just do not understand why other drivers are allowed on the roads when I want them to myself. The worst are cyclists, wobbling about all over the place, ignoring traffic lights, taking up the space of a ten-ton truck. There should be cemented areas for cyclists that are nothing to do with roads at all. Let them circle endlessly in some cyclist-hell. I see that idiot, David Cameron, the wafer-thin (mentally) leader of the Tories, cycles. Put him out to pasture too, I say. At Sir Michael and Lady Shakira's (nothing wrong with a bit of formality) I ate some corncake things with a Pimms. Marvellous lamb with new potatoes, veggies and then far too much Häagen-Dazs vanilla ice cream (Shakira put the carton, with a spoon in it, right in front of me!) and a plum crumble. Later some other cookie things. Long walk in the grounds. Dinner:

apple and carrot juice mixed, a small amount of water biscuit and butter. Night weight 79.3kg.

MONDAY 18 SEPTEMBER
Morning weight 78.5kg or 12st 5lbs. A half-pound increase. Even though I had a very tiny dinner. But this shows you can eat a fairly normal lunch, just not a total pig lunch. At this weight I'm two pounds over my new comfort zone. It will be dealt with. That's the sort of determination we dieters (I hope I can now include you!) must exhibit – and carry out! Breakfast: sheep's milk yoghurt, jam, clementine juice. 10.15am (bit early, please note): coffee with Cadbury's chocolate powder in it plus single malt Scotch and crystal sugar. Lunch: grilled sole, beans, corn on the cob off the cob with butter. Then went to the attic with some assistants and found seven jackets, nine silk shirts and one suit, all fitting me brilliantly! The joys of dieting! 4pm-ish: repeat of the coffee-Scotch-chocolate. Dinner, a problem. Should have had just veggie juice. But it was Dinah May's birthday. First we had some champagne and nuts at home on the terrace. Then Dinah, Geraldine and I went to The Wolseley, where I had 200 grams of Beluga caviar with one small blini and a tiny bit of toast. Wolseley boss, Jeremy King, brought a propped-up macaroon with a birthday message for Dinah in solid icing leaning against it. The macaroon, with chocolate attached, was so good I ate most of it, and then a sliver of Dinah's cheese, and some pink champagne. This was not an enormous meal, but too big. Dieters cannot eat too much, except very occasionally, in the evening. We shall see the damage. Night weight 78.6kg.

TUESDAY 19 SEPTEMBER

Morning weight 78.6kg or 12st 5¼lbs. I'm creeping up a quarter of a pound a day. Not good. Shouldn't have had that chocolate macaroon last night! Greater willpower is called for. 11-ish: coffee-chocolate-Scotch-sugar. Lunch at Cecconi with Paola, Dinah, my assistant, and Joanna Kanska, ex-TV star (*Capital City* etc.), who also works for me. Started with a sort of thick baguette. I had two with ham and one with some veggie paste. Then spaghetti with tomato sauce and other more glam stuff, then bit of plum pud and some other tart. Small espresso. Not a diet meal. PM: coffee-plus again. At 6.30pm: dinner of veggie juice, one small choccy biscuit and some raisins. Night weight a horrific 79.8kg.

WEDNESDAY 20 SEPTEMBER

Morning weight 78.9kg or 12st 6lbs. I am creeping up! You cannot eat a lot of very large and fattening lunches and expect to get away with it, even if you cut back in the evening. The key to this diet is 'Eat less'. For the last six lunches I have not eaten less, I have eaten big-time piggie. This has to stop! Breakfast: usual sheep's milk yoghurt, jam, clementine juice. 11-ish: usual coffee-chocolate-sugar-milk-Scotch. Lunch: a kipper and ratatouille. Before dinner, some Krug champagne with Geraldine, Dinah and my long-time assistant John Fraser MA (Oxon), M.Phil. John started working for me when he was 11 and I was 10 at school. He made my bed, cleaned my room and did my communal washing-up – when they called out 'P to Z', to go and stand in the cold to wash the plates and things in wooden washbasins only covered with an open-to-the-weather lean-to, Fraser turned up for me! John told me that the headmaster had said to him, 'It's the power of the purse, John. You're working for a junior boy.' I said, 'What do you want to do?' John said, 'I'll keep taking the money.' And did so for 60 years. He recently retired. Now has a new knee and new hip, but suffers from withered limbs through polio when young. He'd just come out of hospital and nursing home. Thus the champagne and some nuts and raisins. We still use his name writing letters and emails. In fact, he writes more since he left us than he did when he was there in the flesh! John went on to a staff party. I walked in Holland Park with Geraldine. Came back and had freshly made apple, pear and one banana juice! Nothing else! Then at around 10pm Geraldine returned from Fraser's 'do' and brought a bit of white iced cake for me. I foolishly had a few mouthfuls of it. It was not very good. Why did I do that? Because I'm stupid. Night weight 80kg.

THURSDAY 21 SEPTEMBER

Morning weight 79.1kg or 12st 6¼lbs. Disappointing. I ate very little yesterday. Here I am up a quarter of a pound. And yesterday we took from the attic (preserved in plastic but with a moth-hole that will be invisibly mended) a 1988 evening dress that fitted perfectly. In my current wardrobe I have two other evening dresses – one made when I got too fat for the 'attic' one and another made when I got too fat for the one I had made after the 'attic' one, if you get my drift. I cannot put on much more weight. There is a price to staying slim and lovely. Breakfast: sheep's milk yoghurt, jam (maybe I should have cut out the jam?), clementine juice. Lunch at Cecconi again, this time with Roderick Mann, a marvellous ex-journalist, once engaged to Kim Novak, who did show-business interviews funnier and better than anyone has done before or since. He inherited all of his good friend Cary Grant's clothes. Since Cary took everything he could grab, from airline crockery up and down, this included all his famous film suits and jackets. 'Sell them, Roddy,' I advised. He thought it might be vulgar. 'You'll get at least a million dollars,' I expounded. He's thinking about it. I mean, what else is he going to do with them? I ate crostini with ham, sea bream with spinach, and a lemon sorbet plus a Buck's Fizz. It's very buzzy, Cecconi, packed with lots of beautiful people. Sit down the reader who said, 'Then what were you doing there?' 5pm-ish: coffee-chocolate-Scotch-milk-sugar. Dinner: glass of Cos-d'Estournel 1995, grilled salmon, peas. Night weight 79.9kg.

FRIDAY 22 SEPTEMBER
Morning weight 79.1kg or 12st 6¼lbs. Hmmm. Not up. Not down. Not bad. Not good enough. Breakfast: sheep's milk yoghurt, jam, clementine juice. 11-ish: coffee-chocolate-Scotch-milk-sugar. For lunch we were testing a new possibility for housekeeper. Donata, who's been with me six years, is moving on. This lady was called Gloria, a Filipino. Oh dear! Chicken was not well cooked, skin not as crisp as it should be. No real taste. The roast potatoes were pathetic. The apple tart miserable. I said to the agent, 'You shouldn't be offering this woman to your clients as a cook.' Next Tuesday we're trying an Indian

who smiles a lot named Maria. Not the one in *Sound of Music*. Another one. No afternoon coffee! Then I got a new proof of my *Sunday Times* column. The editor had changed things a bit to give 55 more words for the letters section. That's nice. Before dinner a small glass of red wine (Cos-d'Estournel Saint Estèphe 1995). Dinner: nuts and raisins (not many) and one glass of apple and pear juice. Night weight 79.6kg.

SATURDAY 23 SEPTEMBER
Morning weight 78.7kg or 12st 5½lbs. Actually I was 78.6kg for three weigh-ins, then a few seconds later I was 78.7. I normally put the lowest morning weight on the temperamental scales. This time I didn't! I was so thrilled at losing a bit of weight again! Three-quarters of a pound to be exact. Clever me. Difficult day ahead though. Tonight I'm having dinner out with the singer/ musician Chris Rea and his wife. Tomorrow a Michael Caine lunch again. Today visit to a David Hockney exhibition and then lunch at Le Caprice. I had some white bread and butter, a Buck's Fizz and a glass of fresh orange juice. I didn't actually order the glass of orange juice. I simply said to the waiter, 'I'd like fresh orange juice in my Buck's Fizz.' He said, 'Of course it's fresh. We come in at seven in the morning to squeeze it.' I said, 'Orange juice squeezed at seven in the morning is not fresh at 1pm!' The waiter was so carried away by my orange juice request he brought both the Buck's Fizz and a full glass of orange juice. Both were freshly squeezed for me, by which I mean then and there. I continued with duck salad and then haddock (cold – I thought it was

going to be hot!) with quail's eggs and salad. Finally an apple and blackberry jelly with cream. Not exactly a lunch for someone slimming and who has to eat dinner as well! About 6pm: coffee-Scotch-chocolate-milk-sugar. Dinner at the River Café with Chris Rea and his wife Joan. I over-ate. Fried zucchini, steak tartare, tagliolini with tomatoes and something, vanilla pannacotta with strawberries, a drink of crushed strawberries and champagne, which has a name but I can't remember it. Mimosa, maybe? This'll be disaster. Substantial lunch and dinner in one day. Night weight 80.2kg.

SUNDAY 24 SEPTEMBER

Morning weight 79.3kg or 12st 6¾lbs. That's one and a quarter pounds put on through a day of careless eating. You can't expect to keep weight off without some discipline. There's absolutely no point in losing weight and then putting it back on. I must keep saying this to myself again and again. All is not lost! But then, how's this for really stupid?! I was in the kitchen doing my own breakfast because the housekeeper's off. I squeezed a large glass of orange juice and then, after I overdosed on sheep's milk yoghurt, I had a crumpet with lots of butter and marmalade! What a moron! 12-ish: coffee-Scotch-chocolate-milk-sugar. Lunch at Michael Caine's house. A Pimms. A very few unsalted nuts. Roast lamb, Brussels sprouts, two roast potatoes, other veg. Bit of ice cream and an apple and blackberry crumble. Watched the film *Volver* in his cinema. After that a small piece of carrot cake, two biscuits and half a cup of tea, no sugar. At home, sheep's milk yoghurt, little bit of jam, some strawberries, small spoonful of brown granulated sugar. This'll be interesting. Not over-eating but what will it show in the morning? Night weight 80.6kg.

MONDAY 25 SEPTEMBER

Morning weight 79.5kg or 12st 7¼lbs. This is getting ridiculous! Up half a pound when I should be going down! Desperate measures are required. For a start I cut out my little pot of jam with breakfast this morning. So I just had sheep's milk yoghurt and clementine juice. This means I denied myself 42g or one and a half ounces of jam. It's the Wilkin & Sons Ltd of Tiptree Essex small jars I use. They are one and three-quarter inches diameter and the same height! Thought you'd like to know that. They're out until I lose quite a bit of weight. Nor will there be sugar in my two daily coffees. So at 11: Scotch-coffee-chocolate-milk, no sugar. Lunch: grilled sole, corn off the cob, bit of butter slapped on (a mistake!), beans. 4-ish: coffee with usual suspects, no sugar. Dinner: vegetable juice freshly extracted, two small chocolate biscuits, one very small spoonful of peanut butter, small glass of Château Lynch-Bages 1995. If this day of minor deprivation doesn't lose some weight I'll throw myself from the basement window. Night weight 80.8kg.

TUESDAY 26 SEPTEMBER

Morning weight 78.9kg or 12st 6lbs. At last a drop. Breakfast: usual sheep's milk yoghurt, clementine juice but no jam. Morning coffee-Scotch-chocolate, but no sugar. At lunch we were trying out an Indian lady housekeeper. She was asked to do roast potatoes but couldn't. She tried to roast new potatoes, which was ridiculous! Her veggies were okay. Her roast duck was pretty good but the duck was much smaller than usual. Not her fault. We ordered our meat, as we have for years, from R Allen of Mount Street. They were recently taken over. This duck must have died of starvation. Thus I wrote to the new owners. I used to praise R Allen endlessly in my *Sunday Times* column. Their meat was totally superior to any other. Now, I'm not sure. For dessert our new lady did apple pie. The apples were crudely sliced but fine, the so-called pastry rather solid and biscuity. She's a very nice, cheerful woman so she's still in the running. There's no chance she'll win *Master Chef*. PM: no coffee or anything. Dinner: I picked bits off the duck and ate them. Also had some of the apples, but no pastry, from lunch's apple tart. Night weight 79.7kg.

WEDNESDAY 27 SEPTEMBER

Morning weight 78.6kg or 12st 5¼lbs. Good, a bit more off! Breakfast: sheep's milk yoghurt (no jam), clementine juice. The yoghurt was a bit tedious without the jam so I added some of the clementine juice! That cheered it up a bit. If you want to keep weight off you can't have a full, cooked English breakfast (one of the world's great meals!) every day. You have to make a decision. Do you want to look decent and years younger or do you want to be a fat pig? As I was for many, many years. In spite of some food deprivation, I'm definitely happier as a thinnie. Mid-morning: coffee, chocolate, Scotch, no sugar. Lunch, a disaster! It was so good. Trying out another housekeeper. This one worked for Valentino for years. The lamb cutlets and veggies were not troubling, the roast potatoes were good, but the dessert – chocolate mousse with flaked white chocolate on top – was a killer. I ate too much. A teaspoonful would have been too much. But it was all first-rate. She may be unlucky and get the job! PM: coffee, Scotch, chocolate, no sugar. Dinner at E&O in Notting Hill Gate. This is a cheerful (I was going to say 'cheap and cheerful' but the bill was £166 for three people!) place that does fringe Asian food. Very tasty. I took my assistant Dinah and Geraldine – and went bonkers over-ordering. We had edamame, prawn dumplings, spare ribs, date gyozas, crispy pork belly – and that was just for starters. Main course was black cod – expensive at £21.50 a portion excluding 12.5 per cent service, but quite delicious. I don't know why more restaurants don't do it. Also egg rice and choi shoots. Then I – and only me, the ladies had nothing – had for dessert cinnamon doughnuts. A mound of them with two dips to dunk them in. At the last minute Geraldine and Dinah shared the last one from my large portion. If this isn't a weight disaster I know not what will be! Night weight 80.1kg.

THURSDAY 28 SEPTEMBER
Morning weight 79.1kg or 12st 6¼lbs. Up a pound. What do you expect if you eat too much! Breakfast: sheep's milk yoghurt, clementine juice, no jam. 11-ish: coffee-Scotch-chocolate-milk, no sugar. Lunch at Scalini with Paola and my assistant Dinah: some bread and cut up tomato. Tiny bit of Parmesan. Fried calamari. Large orange juice. Spaghetti with meatballs and tomato sauce.

Fried zucchini. Lemon sorbet. Too much. I'm alone tonight as Geraldine's in Milan, so I must be very, very careful. I'm not sure I was! I had two large glasses of apple juice with a tiny bit of pear juice thrown in. All freshly extracted by me! Also a melon, with lemon squeezed on it and with some brown sugar added to the second half of the melon. Plus one small chocolate biscuit. Night weight 80.8kg. That is unbelievable! It's difficult to lose more than 1kg or 2.2lbs overnight. That means I'd be around 12 stone eight pounds tomorrow morning. I can't even think of it! I won't sleep!

FRIDAY 29 SEPTEMBER
Morning weight 79.9kg or 12st 8lbs. Exactly what I predicted last night! Ridiculous! I don't understand why I'm up one and three-quarter pounds when I hardly ate any dinner last night and what I had was consumed at 6.30pm! I assume it's because I've been stuffing myself with abandon at lunch. Breakfast: sheep's milk yoghurt, no jam, clementine juice. 11-ish: coffee, chocolate, Scotch, milk. This is unbelievable. We had another cook-housekeeper from a well-known domestic agency come in to do a trial lunch. She was asked to do apple pie. She said to my assistant Dinah, 'Is there a recipe book here so I can find out how to make pastry?' Then she asked a few more bizarre questions. Finally Dinah said to me, 'There's no point in trying her out!' We've seen one woman from Portugal, who's far and away the best cook. She did lunch last Wednesday. But I think she worked here before. When I asked her she said, 'I can't remember!' She's very temperamental and walked out

last time. Today my last lunch from the current lady was roast chicken, one roast potato, Brussels sprouts, carrots. 5-ish: coffee, milk, Scotch, chocolate. Alterations tailor came yet again. Dinner: some of the chicken from lunch, two tomatoes. Just before bed, quarter of a cup of chocolate and Horlicks with milk and hot water. Night weight 80.4kg.

SATURDAY 30 SEPTEMBER
Morning weight 79.6kg or 12st 7½lbs. At least it's going down! I wonder if I put on weight so much these last few days because Geraldine's in Milan and I'm not doing my one-hour forced walk each evening? Breakfast: sheep's milk yoghurt, no jam, clementine juice. 12-ish: coffee-Scotch-chocolate-milk. Geraldine's plane from Milan was delayed, so she got back at 1pm. By 1.30 we were looking around for a rare 'drop in' lunch. We passed the Notting Hill Brasserie, when Geraldine spotted a parking spot. Pay and display. I parked while she checked we could get in. I put £5 in the machine to get a parking permit only to have Geraldine point out it was after 1.30 so parking was free. Can I get my £5 back from the Kensington and Chelsea Council, I wonder? Pretty good, the Brasserie. Nice big room. Very fine fresh bread roll with olives in it. Freebie starter of sea bream tarted up. Geraldine had sea bass, I had eggs Benedict. To start I had an artichoke soup, to finish a home-made vanilla yoghurt with berries. It was all fine. Not much atmosphere. In fact nil atmosphere. But very good food. Took a one-hour walk. Watched *Meet the Fockers* in my private cinema. Forgot I'd seen it before. But it was very charming. Beautifully

acted. Good bit of Hollywood entertainment. Dinner: glass of water, two very small chocolate biscuits, one apple. Night weight 80kg.

SUNDAY 1 OCTOBER

Morning weight 79kg or 12st 6lbs. One and a half pounds down. A result to celebrate. But an hour after weighing in three times at 79kg, and having done nothing but have a jacuzzi, a swim and walk about, my posh balancing scales put me at 79.1kg. Five minutes later my bathroom scales, which had me at 79kg an hour earlier, put me at 79.4kg! What's a poor girl to think?! Anyway, I always take the lowest morning weight, and then only after standing on the scales and getting it three times. Breakfast: clementine juice, sheep's milk yoghurt and – recklessly – a little brown sugar added to cheer it up. Lunch at the Orrery. This is owned by Terence Conran. My *Sunday Times* column started with a single article written to get revenge on Terence for a dismissive letter he sent me in reply to a horrible experience at his Pont de la Tour restaurant. He wrote and spoke rudely about me for years. I spoke and wrote rudely about him. Then I went over to him at the pool of the Cipriani in Venice. He thought I was going to make a scene. But we became friends and that night his wife rang to ask if I could use my influence at Harry's Bar to get them a seat in the ground-floor bar area, because he couldn't get one. I got him the table downstairs. We dined some years ago at his Almeida restaurant in Islington (very good) and planned further meetings but never had any. At the Orrery I was with Roderick Mann, whom I'd taken to Cecconi's. I had a small baguette, a Buck's Fizz, a freebie starter of smoked salmon jelly with cauliflower foam. Then some foie gras and a brioche. Main course, a saffron risotto, baby asparagus and broad beans. Also some of Geraldine's duck. A terrible dessert of peanut butter parfait, bitter chocolate ganache and cream. It was ghastly and very cloying. Rest was good. Then a couple of petit fours and an espresso coffee. Big meal, piggy meal. But I intend to have no dinner. Watched *Willy Wonka and the Chocolate Factory* in my private cinema. Very important when you don't want to eat to have something to distract you! Afterwards had one sheep's milk yoghurt with jam. Night weight 80.3kg.

MONDAY 2 OCTOBER
Morning weight 79.3kg or 12st 6 ¾lbs. I'm really surprised I've put on three-quarters of a pound after basically no dinner last night. Must have been that dreadful, heavy dessert at the Orrery yesterday. Oh well. Onwards and downwards! I had my usual breakfast of sheep's milk yoghurt and clementine juice. 11-ish: coffee, Scotch, chocolate, milk. Lunch with Laurel Powers-Freeling, head of American Express in the UK. Laurel plays the harpsichord. Very well! She chose Joël Robuchon's restaurant next to The Ivy. He wasn't actually there, M. Robuchon, nor is he very much. We went upstairs to the posher bit of it, atrociously designed and laid out, which is called La Cuisine. Very good food. I ate far, far, far too much. Started with carta da musica crisp Italian bread. A bit of a baguette (quite awful!) and then a little freebie starter of mousse of foie gras topped with a reduction of

port served with a froth of Parmesan. Also some excellent Spanish ham. Then three fried langoustines. Then, not ordered, two scallops baked in the open-fired oven and served with a citrus and seaweed butter. Main course was roasted young duck, orange jus and endives plus some mashed potato. Dessert was crispy meringue, lemon and lime sorbet, avocado banana. Small but good. Then they gave us a digestif of peach liqueur with raspberries on top. Plus an espresso coffee – plus a Buck's Fizz, plus a glass of red wine (2002 Geyersville Ridge Vineyard Santa Cruz USA). That is not on any normal diet. I will not eat tonight to make up for it! I didn't even have my usual coffee in the afternoon. Well, just a tiny sip of a tiny bit. I want to be 12 stone three pounds. I'm some three pounds over. But I'm not unhappy because I'm a helluva lot less than 15 stone 10 pounds, which I was for years! Dinner was – wait for it – a glass of Malvern still mineral water with some fresh lemon squeezed into it. Absolutely nothing else! That after a one-hour walk! In order not to feel tempted to eat it's useful to be stuck in my cinema, so we ran *Elizabethtown*, a 123-minute movie with Orlando Bloom, Kirsten Dunst and Susan Sarandon. Quite good. Passed the time, and when I came out at 10.30pm I wasn't that hungry. This is the sort of thing you'll have to do occasionally if you want to keep weight off. Won't kill you, I promise! The extra weight might! Night weight 80.2kg.

TUESDAY 3 OCTOBER

Morning weight 79.3kg or 12st 6¾lbs. That is very disappointing after only having a glass of water for dinner last night. Weight same as yesterday morning.

Some people say weight loss isn't shown by what you eat the day before. It takes 48 hours. In which case, tomorrow I expect to be light as a feather. So thin I'll be invisible. Breakfast: sheep's milk yoghurt, clementine juice. We're trying out this Indian lady cook-housekeeper again today. She's always smiling. That's a major plus. I said, 'What desserts can you do?' She replied, 'Rice pudding.' I asked, 'Is that it?' She smiled. I told her to get some golden syrup to go with the rice pudding. Add cream as well and you have one of the great puddings of the world. Anyone on a diet would ask for golden syrup, wouldn't they? So for lunch I had grilled sole with string beans and asparagus, then rice pudding with golden syrup and cream. 5-ish: coffee-chocolate-Scotch-milk. Went to two 'parties'. First to Claridge's ballroom, where Gordon Ramsay was hosting a launch for his auto-biography. Gordon famously phoned me one night at 6.30 as I was having dinner in the kitchen and said, 'Whatever the *Daily Telegraph* claims I said tomorrow, I didn't.' So, of course, I knew Gordon had shot his mouth off, was having regrets and felt a certain degree of fear at upsetting me. The next day he was quoted saying, 'Michael Winner knows nothing about food.' The *Telegraph* rang me for a response. 'God, the truth hurts,' I said. I'm a great fan of Gordon. We've had a few spats, but so what! I always go to his 'do's' to support him. At this one I had five excellent canapés. The second event was a party stated as being to celebrate 25 years of Le Caprice. Since I frequented the Caprice in the early 1950s I couldn't quite see where 25 years came in. It was actually from the re-birth with Jeremy King and

Christopher Corbin, neither of whom chose to turn up! This was at the Serpentine Gallery. A daft place for a party in what could have been severe rain, though lucky for the organisers there was just some drizzle. You had to walk quite a way to get to the entrance. Then there was an open area between the old building Serpentine Gallery and the new 'balloon', which is another large room. Had it rained, all the guests would have been soaked. I had one canapé there. Didn't see many anyway. The one I had was not a patch on the ones at Claridge's. Back home I had a few strawberries and raspberries, no sugar or anything. Night weight 79.8kg.

WEDNESDAY 4 OCTOBER
Morning weight 79kg or 12st 6lbs. At least I lost three-quarters of a pound. Breakfast: sheep's milk yoghurt (onto which I sneaked a little brown granulated sugar), clementine juice. 11-ish: usual coffee-Scotch-chocolate-milk. Lunch was another test for our Indian possible-cook-housekeeper. She did chicken curry. Absolutely superb. I ate much too much, rice, veggies, all that. No dessert. Also new PA started today. We had a drama last week. My Olympus machine that plays back mini-tapes from my recorder collapsed. I tape-record things on all my trips and meals for the *Sunday Times* and do all my letters on these little cassette recorders. We couldn't find a replacement playback machine in the High Street. On the internet all the playback machines are now digital. The Chief Executive of Olympus said he was sure they'd find my now-extinct machine somewhere. But they didn't. This new PA, Rose, located one, before she even joined us, on sale in a second-

hand shop in Glasgow. I know not how because she lives in Kent! So in theory they're sending two, which we'll get tomorrow! 6pm-ish: coffee-chocolate-Scotch-milk. Dinner: very thick Brie cheese and tomato toasted sandwich with fresh vegetable juice. Night weight 80kg.

THURSDAY 5 OCTOBER

Morning weight 79kg or 12st 6lbs. No rise, no fall. Good, but not good enough. I am not achieving exactly what I want to achieve. But then, who does? Breakfast: I went mad and added a little pot of jam to my sheep's milk yoghurt. Also drank clementine juice. 10am (please note a bit earlier than usual!): coffee-Scotch-chocolate-milk. Dinah helped the Indian lady with the lunch because she didn't know how to do roast potatoes or Yorkshire pudding. It turned out pretty well. I had roast beef, Yorkshire pudding (which could have been a bit crisper), three roast potatoes (which were excellent) and some veggies. Quite a big meal really. 4pm-ish: usual coffee plus drink! My Olympus mini-cassette transcribing machine did not arrive! That's Parcel Force for you. PF online said it was 'on the way'. What a shambles they are. Went to opening of Charles Saatchi's USA exhibition at the Royal Academy. Jolly. Drank nothing. Had one bite of a breadstick dipped in cream cheese. Home to eat a tomato and blue cheese sandwich, some freshly extracted vegetable juice and then some cashew nuts unsalted. Problem was this was later than usual. Finished about 9.45pm. Normally eat at 6.30pm. This will do no good eating and going to bed within a couple of hours. Oh dear. Night weight 79.7kg.

FRIDAY 6 OCTOBER
Morning weight 78.9kg or 12st 6lbs. Can't seem to get away from 12 stone six pounds. Greater effort is needed. Not terrible, really, when I was satisfied with 12 stone 12 pounds to 13 stone two pounds as my 'resting' weight. Breakfast: sheep's milk yoghurt, little brown granulated sugar with it, clementine juice. Lunch: a rather failed chicken soup from our trial cook. Dinah said the bones needed boiling for two and half hours at least. But the chicken itself with rice and veggies was good. Some red wine 6pm-ish. More trouble from Parcel Force. They have no force whatsoever. Their printout per their internet site was rubbish. We're still awaiting delivery of something sent two days ago. I located Lynn Gawthorpe, who had the grand title Chairman's Office Adviser for Parcel Force. She confirmed the computer printout we got was a lie. They had not, as claimed, tried to deliver my machine on Thursday, but they would today without fail. They didn't! At 5pm she said, 'I've spoken to the local branch and they promise me it will be delivered tomorrow before 12 noon.' We'll see. A walk. Dinner: a chicken and tomato toasted sandwich with mayonnaise. A few nuts. Night weight 79.6kg.

SATURDAY 7 OCTOBER
Morning weight 78.7kg or 12st 5½lbs At last! I've lost half a pound! Breakfast: sheep's milk yoghurt with some brown granulated sugar, clementine juice. 11-ish: coffee-choc-Scotch-milk. 12 noon and my promised (again) cassette player has not arrived! Lunch at The Ivy. I mistakenly told my guest, Roderick Mann, to meet me at

Le Caprice. He was none too pleased to find I wasn't there! As he took a taxi-ride to The Ivy, it gave me a chance to walk next door to L'Atelier Robuchon, where I'd lunched on Monday. The downstairs, which newspapers said was so popular you had to queue, was far from full. The manager told me the upstairs restaurant was more or less empty. Journalists write that you have to book three months in advance! At The Ivy, which was packed, I had the set lunch – £25.75 for three courses (£2 less if you eat at a table in the bar) – and very good it was. I had a Buck's Fizz, a tiny bit of white wine and, to eat, crispy pork and honeyed parsnip salad, then braised short ribs of beef with champ and glazed carrots, followed by baked greengage and custard tart. Plus some bread and butter, plus an espresso coffee. Walk in park. Called my hired car driver, Alan, at 6.45pm and said, 'Are you outside the house?' He said, 'I'm at home. You never booked me!' So in one day I gave my lunch guest the wrong restaurant and also forgot I hadn't booked the chauffeur car! Would you say this is a sign of old age, moron-life approaching, or just forgetting as we all do sometimes? Dinner: a glass of freshly made apple juice. Then I drove to the theatre and parked without a problem. Thus saving about £300! Saw the big US musical *Wicked*. Pretty good. No melodies anywhere. They'd have helped! Back home had half a Twix bar and a glass of water to go with my Metformin pill. Silly. Choccie bar was not necessary! Night weight 79.7kg.

SUNDAY 8 OCTOBER
Morning weight 78.8kg or 12st 5¾lbs. Quarter of a pound up! And dinner was only apple juice and later half a Twix

bar! I didn't even like the Twix bar! But it's like alcoholics who go to Alcoholics Anonymous. Piggy-people – them what stuff themselves – are always pigs, even if they're cured pigs. Old habits die hard. Like me eating the Twix bar. Still, I was 13 stone three pounds on 5 July. So things are still vaguely under control. I had my usual breakfast of sheep's milk yoghurt and clementine juice. 12-ish: coffee-Scotch-chocolate-milk. Too much lunch at the River Café: fried zucchini, pumpkin and onions and sage leaves, then bruschetta, Buck's Fizz made with orange juice squeezed then and there, not earlier. Tagliolini with crabmeat. Pheasant with cherries. A brilliant vanilla pannacotta with tiny berries. Dinner: glass of freshly made apple juice. Watched a movie in my home cinema – *Lucky Number Slevin*. Bloody good! Night weight 80.2kg.

MONDAY 9 OCTOBER

Morning weight 79.1kg or 12st 6¼lbs. Up half a pound with only apple juice for dinner! The key to losing weight and keeping it off is: eat less. I am not eating less these days when it comes to lunch. I'm eating enormously. Don't do as I do. Do as I say. I'll have to take that lesson on board myself. If you want to be slim and stay slim you can't eat a gargantuan lunch regularly! I am still well down in weight, but not quite enough. I'm still three and a quarter pounds off my ideal weight. How will I get there? Let's see! After my usual breakfast, this morning I went into quiet but biting rage at Lynn Gawthorpe of Parcel Force. 'I may as well talk to the check-out girl in my local Tesco's,' I said. 'You just promise everything and nothing gets done. Yet again there is no sign of my parcel posted last Wednesday that should have been here on Thursday.' 'I can only apologise,' said Ms Gawthorpe, 'the local manager let me down.' 'Let me explain something,' I said. 'If this parcel is not with me today I am issuing a writ for damages against Parcel Force, which will immediately be reported in the press. Even if I don't get damages the court case will be a publicity disaster for Parcel Force. You will be asked to attend and the promises you've made will be offered as evidence of incompetence. Enough is enough.' At last, late morning, the package arrived. Parcel Force is, without doubt, the most pathetic organisation I've come across in nearly 71 years of half-life! 11-ish: coffee-chocolate-Scotch-milk. Lunch provided by my 'on trial' Indian cook-house-keeper: lamb curry, rice, two veggies Indian style. Very, very good. I had a large first portion and then took a large second portion! Dinner: one glass of apple juice, freshly extracted. One very small chocolate biscuit. Walk in park for an hour. I felt no hunger pangs whatsoever. That's what happens – you get used to not eating dinner. Unbelievable for a pig like me! Night weight 80.3kg.

TUESDAY 10 OCTOBER
Morning weight 79.3kg or 12st 6¾lbs. Question: How can you put on half a pound when you only have apple juice for dinner! Answer: Very easily if you eat too much lunch. Breakfast: sheep's milk yoghurt with granulated brown sugar, clementine juice. 11-ish: coffee-chocolate-Scotch-milk. Lunch at The Wolseley with Paola. We're planning her birthday party in early November. Last year we had to

cancel because that's when it was found she had cancer and had both breasts removed. Before that she'd had a cyst taken out of her ovaries. After the cancer she had her ovaries out to stop oestrogen production, which can cause further cancer. She's dealt with all that and further complications with immense fortitude. I, on the other hand, pigged out again. I think I need psychological help! Started with smoked salmon and small piece of brown bread, then roast duck in orange with some mashed potato and beans, and then – the killer – some sort of ice cream and whipped cream and a lot of other fat-producing extras. I think it was some sort of caramel coupe. Felt stuffed. I'll have to cut down on the apple juice for dinner. In fact had half a glass of apple juice, then a walk in Holland Park for an hour, then half a glass of vegetable juice and some unsalted almonds. Night weight – this is a laugh! At 10pm I went up to my very large studio bed-sitting room. I weighed myself. I was 79.5kg. Whoopee! About one pound lighter than last night. Then I watched telly and an hour later I weighed myself again. I was now 79.9kg. Nearly a pound heavier. I hadn't eaten anything. I was just sitting. I weighed myself 10 minutes later and I was up to 80kg. Work that out!

WEDNESDAY 11 OCTOBER
Morning weight 79kg or 12st 6lbs. A loss of three-quarters of a pound. At last! Breakfast: sheep's milk yoghurt with granulated brown sugar, clementine juice. 11-ish: Scotch-coffee-chocolate-milk. Lunch: another try-out of our Indian lady. Roast chicken with roast potatoes, fresh vegetables. She's certainly got the roast potatoes

right. I had three bits, not full potatoes of course. Then she made some rather odd Indian cake that I hadn't asked for. Usually just have a one-course lunch. The cake needed whipped fresh cream, but luckily it wasn't there or I'd have eaten more. Another transport drama – ordered a car from a car service as it was my chauffeur's day off. They rang when it was meant to be here to say as it was Ramadan they'd be very late. So I drove myself to Andrew Neil's bash for *The Business* magazine at the ghastly Mandarin Oriental hotel in Knightsbridge. Before going had some cold chicken from lunch, a glass of freshly extracted apple juice and a tiny bit of cake from lunch. At Andrew's 'do' had one marshmallow (pink, not white!) and three little strips of crystallised orange peel. 11.30pm: hot chocolate-Horlicks-milk-water-little brown sugar. Night weight 79.3kg.

THURSDAY 12 OCTOBER

Morning weight 78.6kg or 12st 5¼lbs. Persistence pays off! Down another three-quarters of a pound. Breakfast: sheep's milk yoghurt with a little brown sugar, clementine juice. Lunch (still trying out this Indian lady): overcooked sea bass (I left most of it), OK broccoli (God, how I hate broccoli!) and corn off the cob. Dinner started with half a glass of freshly extracted vegetable juice. Then, out for the second night running, rare for me, to Kensington Place, where foodie Tom Parker Bowles was launching his new book. I like him. People I like, which aren't many, I always turn up to support. Very crowded. Had two cheese straws and a sliver of crispy bacon. Said 'hello' and had a brief chat with Tom and his mother Camilla. Very nice woman. Also spent time with my all-time favourite chef, Simon Hopkinson, who opened, and used to cook at, Bibendum. But a long time ago, after seven years in the kitchen, Simon quit. On our way out we got two goodie bags, presents given by those hoping you'll later buy their products. This was a bit disastrous. One container had Duchy organic cheese nibbles with mustard. I ate far too many of those. I was only going to have apple juice. Then there was a plastic bottle of blackcurrant and gooseberry smoothie. I drank that. More than enough! Night weight 79.1kg.

FRIDAY 13 OCTOBER
Morning weight 78.1kg or 12st 4¼lbs. Another pound down. That's probably because I ate hardly any lunch yesterday, even though I ate a tiny bit more than I should have for dinner. Breakfast: sheep's milk yoghurt with granulated brown sugar, clementine juice. 11-ish: coffee-chocolate-milk-Scotch. Lunch, with Indian testing-housekeeper: very good roast pork (she got the crackling really crackling), roast potatoes, asparagus. My two Filipino cleaners seem to think I should hire a Filipino cook-housekeeper. I've tried out two of those. They were hopeless. Seen many. I used to have an Irish woman and a Welsh woman who did the job that three people do now. Every time I gave the Welsh lady a salary rise she said, 'I don't know why you've given me this. I haven't done anything for it!' Those days are over! They were both brilliant. The Irish lady did a hot chocolate pud with chocolate sauce and whipped cream that Sophia Loren adored. As did I. Sadly, if not tragically, they both retired.

Today the available menu is somewhat limited! I'll test a couple of new contenders next week, then I'll have to make a choice. Dinner: little bit of Gruyère cheese, some (not much) water biscuit and butter, half a glass of vegetable juice, a third of a Twix bar, eight salted peanuts. 11.30pm: hot chocolate-Horlicks with a tiny bit of brown sugar. Night weight 78.9kg.

SATURDAY 14 OCTOBER

Morning weight 77.9kg or 12st 3¾lbs. Good. Down another half a pound. Breakfast: sheep's milk yoghurt with brown granulated sugar, clementine juice. 11-ish: coffee-chocolate-milk-Scotch. Lunch at a place I've been meaning to visit for years, a very quaint little restaurant in Campden Hill called The Kandy Tea Room. It looks like something out of yesteryear. You imagine it owned by two old ladies, like the faded British that used to inhabit Kensington, staying over from days gone by. In fact it's run and owned by a charming man from Ceylon (now Sri Lanka). I had a toasted cheese and tomato thingy on their home-made bread with a salad, and Geraldine an egg mayonnaise sandwich, smoked salmon and salad. I nicked some of her sandwich. I had Earl Grey tea, chocolate cake – or a bit of it – and a small piece of apple pie, which was fairly awful. Then a scone. Best ever – but should have been served warm. With jam and clotted cream of course. Then I went to a wonderful old church in the East End where they sell stuff from old mansions, period ironmongery, fireplaces, whatever. This was followed by a real test – Roger Moore's 79th-birthday party at Annabel's. We were asked not to get there until

9pm. It's the worst to eat late, eat too much and then go to bed. I switched my mind to a gear of total determination. I told the Annabel's staff that when I came in they should tell the chef not to worry if I hardly ate anything. It was because I was on this diet. The first food I was offered was in the bar: large prawns, grilled with pepper. They were so good I ate two. Then we went into the private dining room. I don't go to Annabel's much. It has been 'the' place for decades. Used to be a bit stuffy. Now it is full of young people, many not even wearing ties. I'd put on a tie and looked unbelievably thin and smart. Everyone commented on how young and how much better I looked. The first course was delicious crab meat. That was all right, not fattening. I ate it. Next course was lamb cutlets with mashed potatoes with carrots decoratively draped on top. I took two cutlets. Declined the mash and carrots. Had some spinach instead. I hate spinach but they did it so well I had seconds. They had some crispbread, kind of like Ryvita, on the table. I had a little bit of that. So far, not bad. Then came the birthday cake. Chocolate. I was sitting next to Sir Roger, on his right. I had to eat the cake, didn't I? No, I didn't. But I did. Not an enormous piece but not tiny either. Nor was there any reason for me to eat the ice cream in a little cup that was served with it. But I did. Nor was there any reason for me to eat a triple macaroon petit four and a chocolate petit four, but I did. Pig habits die hard. At 11.30 we finished eating. By 12.30 I was in bed. 'I'll pay for this,' I thought. But you can't be totally cautious all the time. We dieters have to get a balance. I dreaded weighing myself for my night weight. It was 78.9kg.

SUNDAY 15 OCTOBER

Morning weight 78.4kg or 12st 4¾lbs. Up one pound. And note you don't lose as much at night when you eat late! Ah, well, weight increase was to be expected. I can, and will, pull back from that. Some people say what you eat the day before doesn't affect your weight the next day. I haven't found that to be so. If I eat heavily one day it shows on the scales the next morning. There's nearly a whole page in the *Mail on Sunday* today about how thin I am compared to what I was. There's a photo of me fat on the beach in Barbados and a photo of me (sneaked) walking outside my house, which the *Mail* says shows how thin I've become. In fact I'm wearing a slightly balloonish leather zip-up jacket so I don't think it shows my new sylph-like figure to its best advantage. I could have worn one of my four-times-taken-in jackets and really looked thin! Also interesting to note the paparazzi are staking out my house! My photo in the *Sunday Times* had me looking very thin, but the faces are all too dark. I've mentioned this to them before. When I graded movies, each with about 4,000 different images in them, the key rule was, 'Get the skin tones right'. Not dark. Not too light. But right. I must remind the *Sunday Times* of this yet again! Usual breakfast. Lunch at The Wolseley: Buck's Fizz, some bread and butter, smoked salmon, roast beef, Yorkshire pudding, one roast potato, green beans, apple crumble, vanilla milkshake. Certainly no dinner tonight. Well, three-quarters of a glass of apple juice. Then watched the film *The Three Burials of Melquiades Estrada*, directed and starring Tommy Lee Jones. To which you may say, 'What's that got to do with dieting?'

It has. Because if you're not going to eat it helps to be shut up in a private cinema to take your mind off it. When I came out I had a little Gruyère cheese. Later, a drink of chocolate-Horlicks with a tiny bit of brown sugar, made with milk and mostly water. Night weight 79.4kg.

MONDAY 16 OCTOBER
Morning weight 78.5kg or 12st 5lbs. Quarter of a pound up. I can deal with that. Lunch at Le Caprice with Henry Wyndham, the Chairman of Sotheby's and a particularly delightful man. I had a bit of bread and butter, not much, crispy duck and watercress salad, braised ox cheek with mushroom and celeriac mash, and a jelly with a bit of cream, followed by (rare for me) a single espresso. Michael, my alterations tailor, came with eight more jackets he'd taken in and took nine away for further diminishing. He's narrowing the arms, taking in the body. It's a major job. Some people say, 'Why not just buy new jackets?' Since new Brioni jackets can easily cost £2,500 each and taking in (or letting out) ones I possess costs about £40 a time, I'd rather spend the £40. After my rather large lunch it meant very little dinner. So after a walk in the park I had one glass of apple juice and some unsalted almonds. 11.30pm: chocolate-Horlicks-milk plus hot water and tiny bit of brown granulated sugar. Night weight 79.2kg.

TUESDAY 17 OCTOBER
Morning weight 78.3kg or 12st 4½lbs. Good. Going down. The *Daily Mail* are coming tomorrow, at their request, to do a 'fashion' photo shoot of me in my 1970s and 80s

jackets rescued from the attic, which I am now wearing. Breakfast: sheep's milk yoghurt with jam, clementine juice. 10-ish: coffee-chocolate-milk-Scotch. The Indian lady housekeeper we've been endlessly testing is testing elsewhere today. So I had no one to prepare lunch. On top of that I needed it at 12.30pm as I was going to Elstree to talk to some big group and had to be there at 2pm. Geraldine saved the day. She went to Luscious Organic, my local healthy food store. There she got chickpea soup (awful), vegetable chilli (delicious), brown rice (perfect) and spinach with chickpeas (very good). That was a pleasing meal. Driving through London is a nightmare. In the centre Ken Livingstone has changed nearly all the traffic lights so they stay on red forever and on green for only a few seconds. Traffic is backed up for miles. Going north there were endless road closures and single-lane driving. Where I live they're adding Britain's largest supermarket complex about a mile away, with parking for 3,000 cars. All of which will use the same vastly overcrowded roads we have to suffer now. Doesn't anyone realise you can't keep putting more and more buildings up with no way of getting to and from them? Back home I had, first, coffee with Scotch and chocolate and, later, apple juice and some water biscuits (not many) with marmalade and butter for dinner. Around 11.30pm: chocolate-Horlicks-milk-water. Night weight 78.9kg.

WEDNESDAY 18 OCTOBER

Morning weight 77.9kg or 12st 3¾lbs. That's a good weight. I've now decided my 'proper' weight is 12 stone one pound to 12 stone five pounds; 12 stone three pounds or below is ideal! I'm so conceited (bet that surprised you!) I was going to take Frumil this morning in preparation for the *Daily Mail* photo shoot. Frumil is a water-loss pill. I used to take it before shooting my commercials. You lose about four pounds and pee a lot! Jockeys take it if they need to get down dramatically to be the right weight on the scales. As I'm so low on the scales this morning I won't bother. Breakfast: sheep's milk yoghurt with granulated brown sugar, clementine juice. 9.40am (early!): coffee-chocolate-Scotch-milk. Lunch at Tom's Café in Notting Hill Gate with the Paola and Dinah May. It's a very good place. I had very freshly squeezed orange juice, some bread and butter, then smoky roast tomato, aubergine and chickpea soup. That was quite extraordinarily excellent. Then Parmesan-crusted chicken with potato gratin and green beans. Plus some minced lamb as if in shepherd's pie. Then a lot of cakes, small pieces of each – I tried lemon crunch cake, chocolate biscuit cake, carrot and pineapple cake, iced stem ginger cake and raspberry meringue. Cakes all superb. Meringue okay but not more than that. Then we went next door to 202 Westbourne Grove because Paola liked the coffee there. As we walked back to my Rolls, paparazzi got out of a car and took photos of us, then sped away! Unbelievable! Geraldine knew I was having lunch with Paola – not exactly a major event – so I hope the press don't try and make something of it. In the afternoon I did my major photo fashion shoot for the *Daily Mail* in various ancient clothes I can now wear. Best of them were an Afghan coat with goat's fur and embroidery, which came from the early 1970s, and an astrakhan-collar coat, real actor-laddie type, that came from the 1950s. Dinner: a glass of apple juice at home. Then a brief visit to Ronnie Scott's Club in Soho for Bill Wyman's 70th birthday. There I had two sausages on sticks and three other small canapés of I know not what. I stayed for a very well done and not too long (which is a miracle) video of Bill's life and some good and equally short speeches, then left, rather naughtily, when his band started playing. I think I'm developing flu. I've taken some Oscillococcinum, a miracle French crystal cure from little plastic phials. This usually works. Hope so. 11.30pm: chocolate-Horlicks-milk-water but this time with Manuka honey, which Geraldine says helps fend off colds. Night weight 78.5kg.

THURSDAY 19 OCTOBER
Morning weight 77.8kg or 12st 3½lbs. That's good, innit! Still going down! I'm holding my cold at bay. Breakfast: sheep's milk yoghurt with jam, clementine juice. 11-ish: coffee-chocolate-Scotch-milk. Lunch: testing a new cook-housekeeper, a Filipino. She wore stiletto heels and a split skirt. Was she offering other services, I wondered?! Roast chicken, roast potatoes, three veggies, stuffing, all pretty good. Apple pie a bit heavy and not enough apple. Cream helped it. Still taking Oscillococcinum. They don't sell it in England any more. You can get it on the Continent, certainly in France. Very good against flu. Joan Collins originally recommended it to me. Dinner, with Geraldine and Dinah, at E&O in Notting Hill. I decided I'd only have soup. But the only soup they had was miso soup, which I hate. So all my good intentions

went out the window. I had baby pork spare ribs, prawn dumpling, pork belly, date gyozas and then black cod with egg rice. I'm pathetic. But I shall live to fight another day. Night weight 79.2kg.

FRIDAY 20 OCTOBER

Morning weight 78.3kg or 12st 4½lbs. Up a pound! That's what happens when you have a big lunch and a big dinner. It's bound to show on the scales. Breakfast: sheep's milk yoghurt, brown granulated sugar, clementine juice. For lunch I'm trying out another Filipino cook-housekeeper. She was doing very well with roast duck, roast potatoes, veggies. And then took a dive. She delivered an apple tart that was cold, felt like it had been standing around forever. I asked why it wasn't warm, or preferably hot, and she said she'd put it in the fridge! Like orange juice, pastry degrades every second it hangs about. I pointed out – keeping calm of course – that apple pie or apple tart is best eaten straight from the oven. We're trying her again on Monday. Ooops! No we're not! Dinah just told me our fishmonger has no fresh Dover soles on Monday. So we'll try her Tuesday. Not easy, all this, is it? Feeling a bit exhausted, I headed for the kitchenette outside my bedroom to make coffee-chocolate-Scotch (do I need that!) with milk. Went for my usual one-hour walk in Holland Park. Returned. Had a glass of apple juice and some of the duck left over from lunch. Night weight 78.8kg.

SATURDAY 21 OCTOBER

Morning weight 77.8kg or 12st 3½lbs. Good. Two pages of 'Winner Thinner' in the *Daily Mail*. Seven photos of me. I must remember not to take any notice when photographers endlessly say 'smile'. I look like a crinkled-up moron. Sit down the reader who said, 'So, what's new?' Breakfast: sheep's milk yoghurt with Manuka honey, clementine juice. I've run out of Oscillococcinum. Thus far it's kept my flu at bay. 11-ish: coffee-chocolate-Scotch-milk. Lunch at San Lorenzo in Knightsbridge: after a Buck's Fizz, I had mixed starter of crostini (sort of tomatoes on toast!), fried calamari and thin slivers of salami, then spaghetti with truffles followed by a chocolate ice cream and two chocolate macaroons. Dinner: one glass of apple juice and some almonds. Then went with Geraldine to see *Spamalot* at the Palace Theatre. Exceedingly funny. That's an entertaining show. Met up, by chance, with the great Dame Judi Dench. She said it was a better production than on Broadway. In the interval we went to the lobby together and I bought her and her friends glasses of champagne. Had one myself. Someone came round selling Spam sandwiches. Judi wanted one. So I got it for her and ate a tiny bit. A lot of people came up to me, having seen my *Daily Mail* thin-Win photo spread, and kindly congratulated me on getting thinner. You see, follow what I say and this will happen to you. You will be deluged with compliments. Even better, your enemies will be furious at your new, younger-looking, better-looking self. That must be worth striving for! Then back to my house, where I had a hot chocolate-Horlicks-milk-water-tiny brown sugar. Night weight 78.5kg.

SUNDAY 22 OCTOBER

Morning weight 77.6kg or 12st 3lbs. That's good, innit?
I don't want to lose more than a couple of pounds now.
And that only as a safety margin. Also good, found some
Oscillococcinum in the back of the bedroom fridge. If
you're ever in France buy this. It's a miracle flu
stopper/cure. Breakfast: sheep's milk yoghurt with
Manuka honey and – wait for it! – not clementine juice,
because I couldn't be bothered to squeeze any as the
staff are off on Sunday. So I had a can of 'Wellman high
performance health and vitality for men'. This I'd
acquired in the freebie goodie bag given after Tom
Parker Bowles' recent book launch party! There was a
picture of someone called Mark Foster on the can – he's
apparently a swimmer – saying, 'Like many professional
sportsmen I rely on Wellman to provide nutritional
support for optimum performance.' It then listed
ingredients, including, but not limited to (as they say in
legal documents), niacin, vitamins B6 and B12, zinc,
folic acid, riboflavin... I could go on. Never mind giving
'high performance' and tasting rather dreary, I slept the
entire afternoon! 12-ish: coffee-chocolate-Scotch-milk.
Lunch at The Wolseley, where I ate a bit of roll and
butter, Buck's Fizz, smoked salmon, tiny bit of brown
bread, roast beef, Yorkshire pudding (didn't eat all of it),
one roast potato. When I've had a vanilla milkshake
here before it's been good but a bit thin, so I asked them
to make it thicker. When it arrived, they'd put in extra
ice cream and it was perfect. Then, real pig-time, I had
an apple strudel and cream, although I left half of it. In
the old days I'd easily have eaten all the beef, the

Yorkshire and the strudel. I really think my stomach must have become smaller. Lulu dropped over to chat at The Wolseley. She looks very slim and young. On returning home, an email from Stirling Moss, whom I've never met, saying, 'Congratulations to you on losing so much weight. Susie [presumably his wife!] wants to know how you did it. Did you have to give up the grape?' I responded that I didn't have to give up anything and all would be revealed in my upcoming *Fat Pig Diet* book. As I was in generous mood (and Stirling was one of the heroes of my youth) I offered to send him a copy free. Do hope I remember! Dinner: one glass of pear, apple and clementine juice, all freshly squeezed or extracted. You will, I hope, have noticed that if you have a big-pig lunch, as I did today, you cannot stay slim by also having a big dinner. You don't have to restrict yourself just to a glass of fruit or veggie juice. Some grilled fish with green vegetables would be OK, or a small lamb cutlet with green veg, a salad with smoked salmon... Those sorts of minimal things would do. And the earlier you eat them the better. You will have had your putting-on-weight stuff – ice cream, pastry, potatoes etc. – for lunch. So you can't claim you're seriously deprived. You're limited. There is a difference. 11pm-ish: chocolate-Horlicks-milk-water-tiny brown granulated sugar. Night weight 78.7kg.

MONDAY 23 OCTOBER
Morning weight 77.6kg or 12st 3lbs. Still good. Breakfast: sheep's milk yoghurt, Manuka honey, clementine juice. 11-ish: hot coffee-chocolate-Scotch-milk. No housekeeper-

testing for lunch so Geraldine did it from our local Luscious Organic shop. Vegetable soup too cold so went back for reheating. Then the main course plates weren't hot! She's a wonderful lady, Geraldine – beautiful, a delight – but per-lease keep her (as with all girlfriends) out of the kitchen. Main course was basmati brown rice, vegetable chilli and mung peas with tofu, which sounds quite awful, but was perfectly pleasant. And very healthy. Evening glass of Lynch-Bages 1995. Then to dinner at Assaggi in Notting Hill Gate. Nino Sassu, chef and co-owner, was on duty. I went with Geraldine and Dinah. No walk, which is not good for the weight. And dinner instead of just apple juice. I had crisp Italian bread, tiny bit of real bread, incredible ham, tagliolini with truffles and then vanilla pannacotta with berries. Too much but I didn't feel bloated. Ended with canarino (lemon peel in hot water), which is supposedly very good for digestion. See what damage is done to my weight situation tomorrow! Night weight 78.5kg.

TUESDAY 24 OCTOBER

Morning weight 77.7kg or 12st 3¼lbs. Not bad. Breakfast: sheep's milk yoghurt with Manuka honey, clementine juice. 11-ish: coffee-chocolate-Scotch-milk. For lunch we tried again a Filipino housekeeper who previously did quite well, but failed dreadfully this time. Two big, juicy Dover soles came in. They were reduced to rubber. Her vegetables were okay at best, including two boiled potatoes, which had no flavour. Her banana cake with whipped cream was good. Dinner should have been just apple juice. But I had to leave early, just after 6pm for a

7pm opening night of *Dirty Dancing*. Geraldine was getting ready, leaving me to knock off two pieces of toast, butter and jam plus my coffee-Scotch-chocolate-milk routine. As that was at 5.40pm it might have been all right. Except that at the first night party, after the show, I ate a small piece of fried chicken and one chip (provided by Judi Dench from her packet!). First nights are always the same. You rush to get there by 7pm, when they say the show will start. (This is made more difficult now through Ken Livingstone having fixed all the central London lights in favour of pedestrians.) You get to the theatre at 6.50pm for a 7pm start. And if they start by 7.20pm it's a miracle! Night weight 78kg.

WEDNESDAY 25 OCTOBER

Morning weight 77.2kg or 12st 2¼lbs. Please note I am now more, I repeat more, that three and a half stone down in weight from what I used to be. It's OK, you don't have to pay extra for the book because I've achieved greater weight loss than announced on the cover and in the publicity. Breakfast: sheep's milk yoghurt, Manuka honey, clementine juice. Geraldine got lunch from a local Italian deli. Turkey burger (rather dry and tough), grilled salmon (good), sort of rice stuff, followed by cheesecake. I didn't eat a gross amount! Glass of Château Lynch-Bages 1995. 4-ish: coffee-chocolate-Scotch-milk. I'll tell you how to make coffee. Take freshly ground coffee and spoon some into a mug or cup. Take another cup of the same size and put in your milk, and – in my case – a spoonful of chocolate and a dash of single malt Scotch. Then pour just-boiled water into the cup with the coffee.

Take a small sieve, put it over the cup with the milk and whatever in it, and pour the coffee into this second cup through the sieve. This uses a lot of coffee, but it is definitely, assuredly and infallibly the only way to make really good coffee. It's also very quick! For dinner at 6.15pm I was drinking my apple juice when Geraldine said peanut butter and banana sandwiches were very healthy! Easily led, I took two pieces of matzos (thin water biscuits, quite large) and added butter, peanut butter and banana. 'Was this wise?' I asked myself as we set out on our usual one-hour walk in Holland Park. We'll see. Night weight 78kg.

THURSDAY 26 OCTOBER

Morning weight 77.1kg or 12st 2lbs. So the peanut butter and banana didn't do damage. I'm a quarter of a pound down. But in trouble today. As well as going to Scalini for lunch I've arranged with Paola to go to Morelli's, the ice cream and milkshake counter in Harrods, for dessert! She's up in town again to see doctors about her physical problems and deep depression. Breakfast: sheep's milk yoghurt with jam, clementine juice. 11-ish: coffee-chocolate-Scotch-milk. Lunch at Scalini with Paola and Dinah: bit of bread with tomatoes in olive oil. Few bits of Parmesan cheese. Tagliolini with truffles. A taste of Paola's porcini mushrooms. Then to Morelli's at Harrods (Paola's a fan). There I had a large milkshake. Also tasted some of Morelli's soft ice cream and a bit of Paola's chocolate sundae. All too much really. But very good. Geraldine was at Covent Garden seeing *Coppelia*, so I had to extract my own apple, pear and banana juice for dinner. That was it, a glass and a half of liquid. Quite enough. Night weight 78.1kg.

FRIDAY 27 OCTOBER
Morning weight 77.4kg or 12st 2½lbs. Lear-jetted to Lisbon. Ate some crisps on the flight! At the Lapa Palace hotel in Lisbon met John Malkovich in the lobby. He was staying there and I'd just booked for lunch at a restaurant he has a share of. It's a sporty sort of place on the water called Bica do Sapato. I had crispy goat's cheese with roast tomato, which took forever to arrive but was very tasty. Then fresh cod poached in olive oil and some salsafine. For dinner at the hotel the general manager recommended, as being typically Portuguese, roast suckling pig. This was excellent but came with totally cold mashed potatoes and some warm cooked onions. Before that they brought tiny portions of foie gras with toast, then sea bass ravioli with tarragon vinaigrette. Dessert was lemon sorbet and some petits fours. Night weight 77.6kg.

SATURDAY 28 OCTOBER
Morning weight 76.7kg or 12st 1lb. I don't believe this! The hotel scales are over-generous. Breakfast was orange juice, freshly squeezed at the table on our terrace in boiling hot sun, a bowl of raspberries and other berries, croissant with butter and jam, a cappuccino, a plain yoghurt with a small amount of granulated sugar. Drove to Sintra, a preserved old village. Lunch at Hockey Caffee there. Fresh orange juice, a few chips that they wanted me to try, goat's cheese and breadsticks, cod on a bed of

spinach with some small baked potatoes, then crêpes with ice cream and cream, which the restaurant manager assured me was fresh, but which I thought came from a squidgy plastic thing. Dinner at the hotel: a little artichoke soup as a freebie starter, Buck's Fizz, poached egg, mushroom and truffles, then tagliolini and truffles, then a lemon sorbet and three petits fours. All too much for a late dinner. Night weight 77.5kg.

SUNDAY 29 OCTOBER

Morning weight 76.7kg or 12st 1lb. Again. I don't believe this! I think the hotel scales are unbelievably kind. Breakfast was berries, ordinary yoghurt, a croissant with jam and butter. It was 80 degrees Fahrenheit so we sunlounged by the pool. Lunch at the hotel started with the heaviest, the most uneatable terrine of veal liver Venetian style and foie gras. It was heavy and clammy. The hotel general manager said he'd just eaten some and found it awful, too. 'I'm taking it off the menu,' he said. Bit late that. Why was it ever on? Dinner at Alcantara Café. Very good open design, as if in an old warehouse with iron pillars. The bread was rubbery. Fresh orange juice. Parmesan millefeuille with smoked salmon and artichoke purée and olive tapenade. Then a bean stew with shellfish and white rice. Dessert was lemon sorbet. The place looked better than the food tasted, but it was okay. Night weight 78.5kg.

MONDAY 30 OCTOBER

My birthday. I'm too old for birthdays. Morning weight 77.6kg or 12st 3lbs. The hotel brought a chocolate birthday cake up at breakfast time on the terrace, where it was 85 degrees Fahrenheit! I took a bit. It was exceptionally good! Then I had a bit of croissant and jam, orange juice, berries and natural Activia yoghurt. We took a drive to a place called Obidos. A preserved village, very white. Not horrible, but not a patch on villages in France such as St Paul de Vence or in Italy such as Apricale. We lunched at the Lidador Café, where they got all the orders wrong. They brought scrambled eggs and sausages, thinking they were for Geraldine, when she'd ordered a prawn cocktail. I got the sausages. Awful. When I said, 'For madame the fish', the owner asked, 'What fish?' I said, 'The one we ordered!' Oh forget it. Portugal is no place for food. Dinner in the Lapa Palace hotel. Some breadsticks, a stuffed zucchini flower, lasagne with wild mushrooms and cheese sauce. On the first day I'd asked the restaurant manager to put the Evian water in an ice bucket. Now, four days later, it still sat, nowhere near ice, on a side table. I did give him a bit of a blast! And what top-class hotel serves Evian in plastic bottles in a grand dining room? The hotel general manager had recommended crème brûlée for dessert with truffles. He made a big thing about the fact they did it with truffles. When the dessert came there was no sign of truffles. 'They don't know what they're doing here,' observed Geraldine. Very true. Night weight 79kg.

TUESDAY 31 OCTOBER
Morning weight 78kg or 12st 4lbs. Last weight on hotel scales. It'll be interesting to see what my normal scales have to say on this highly important matter! Breakfast:

berries, some sort of roll with jam and butter, no yoghurt, coffee. Then to a teeny weenie little private jet called a Cessna 1. Held up by fog at Lisbon airport! On the plane I ate a rather clammy white bread smoked salmon sandwich (half a piece of bread) and some sort of paste sandwich and drank Evian. Dinner at home was apple juice, some water biscuits with butter and jam, and hazelnuts with raisins. One-hour walk, to hopefully get some weight off. Later a chocolate and Horlicks drink. Night weight a mildly horrifying 79.4kg

WEDNESDAY 1 NOVEMBER
Morning weight 78.8kg or 12st 5¾lbs. As I feared, the hotel scales were rather complimentary. My target weight zone is 12 stone two pounds to 12 stone five pounds. So I'm a bit over. Breakfast: sheep's milk yoghurt, jam, clementine juice. 11-ish: coffee-chocolate-Scotch-milk. Lunch: re-testing a Filipino housekeeper who turned sole into rubber last time. This time she tried again. It wasn't rubber, but nor was it historic. Various veggies, no potatoes. Then a rhubarb and raspberry tart with whipped cream. That was good but didn't really speak volumes! In fact, none of the food tasted of much. No pizzazz! A Portuguese housekeeper, whom I once employed and who walked out on me, wants to come back. She's moving into pole position! Dinner was apple juice and a few hazelnuts. Walked 7 to 8pm. Then off to a party given in a club in St James's Square opposite my memorial to PC Yvonne Fletcher. It was to celebrate 30 years of Britain's top literary agent, Ed Victor. Very posh crowd. I declined all food and drink. When Lord Andrew

Lloyd Webber and his wife Madeleine asked me to have dinner with them I said, 'I can't eat! I've had my apple juice! But I'll sit and smile.' They decided to skip dinner and go back to the dress rehearsal of *The Sound of Music*. I went home, congratulating myself on my extraordinary abstinence. You wanna stay thin, that's what you have to do. You wanna be a fat pig, don't. Night weight 79.2kg.

THURSDAY 2 NOVEMBER
Morning weight 78.4kg or 12st 4¾lbs. On the way down! Breakfast: sheep's milk yoghurt, jam, clementine juice. 11-ish: coffee-chocolate-Scotch-milk. Lunch was to be another test of yesterday's housekeeper but she's ill! So Geraldine got a shepherd's pie and a cottage pie from our local butcher, Lidgate, and she did some salad. 4-ish: coffee-chocolate-Scotch-milk. Dinner, very cautious: apple juice and water biscuits, jam and butter. One-hour walk. Tailor brought back 17 taken-in jackets, many for the sixth time! And seven pairs of trousers taken in at waist and thigh! Takes hours to put them away properly. They all have to be labelled so I know what fits and what still needs attention! I need a butler. No, three butlers. And a clothes filing clerk. Night weight 78.4kg.

FRIDAY 3 NOVEMBER
Morning weight 77.5kg or 12st 2¾lbs. Good. It's little weight-loss triumphs like this that keep us dieters going. I don't want to go below 12 stone. Not that this is likely! I have to be ever vigilant to stay approximately where I am. Breakfast: sheep's milk yoghurt, jam, clementine juice. 11-ish: coffee-chocolate-Scotch-milk. Lunch at The

Wolseley, which gets better and better. Smoked salmon, caviar omelette with double portion of caviar, two bread rolls because today they came heated (unusual) and they have very good butter. Dessert, a vanilla milkshake. Since I persuaded them to add extra ice cream to the milkshakes they really are superb. And a tiny bit of banana cake as ordered by the Paola. Before dinner went to the Dorchester to a reception for Leslie Pound, a marvellous 80-year-old public relations man working for one of Britain's major film distributors. He was to retire at the end of the year. Nice to meet and chat with Dickie Attenborough and director Lewis Gilbert. 'God they look old!' I ungraciously thought. Had one small smoked salmon canapé. Dinner: apple juice, and a small birthday cake I'd forgotten about. Fruitcake it was, with white icing. Just before bed, a tiny sliver of bread and butter because I'd forgotten to take my Metformin pill and milk thistle pill, and you're meant to have something in the stomach with them. Night weight 78.3kg.

SATURDAY 4 NOVEMBER

Morning weight 77.5kg or 12st 2¾lbs. Good. Breakfast: sheep's milk yoghurt, jam, clementine juice. 11-ish: coffee-chocolate-Scotch-milk. Lunch at The Ivy. Their set lunch is spectacularly good value. I had a Buck's Fizz, a white bread roll with butter, then cep tart with goat's cheese sauce, veal and ham meatballs with borlotti beans, and a hot chocolate sponge pudding with custard. You don't see many 'faces' in The Ivy at Saturday lunch. Just a jolly group of people who probably booked months ahead. But my old friend, director John Boorman, was there. He got his first feature movie when I left (for something better) on pre-production of *Catch Us If You Can* with the Dave Clark Five, an early Sixties pop band. John took over and carved a great career out of it. For dinner I was driven to Epsom. I didn't know people lived there. I thought it was just for horses. But my commercials' employer, Peter Wood, chairman of the insurance group esure, was giving his 60th-birthday bash in an enormous marquee in his garden. I ate not much, being careful – little smoked salmon, chicken, apple crumble. Had nothing to drink but Evian water. Night weight 79kg.

SUNDAY 5 NOVEMBER

Morning weight 77.7kg or 12st 3¼lbs. Because I ate in the evening – not much but more than I should have – I'm up half a pound. Breakfast as usual. 12-ish: coffee-chocolate-Scotch-milk. Lunch at home: Geraldine got some steak from Waitrose. Not my normal quality of supplier by a long way. Then I overcooked it. She did a good salad with an egg mayonnaise, plus some smoked salmon from our local organic shop, which was very good. We've been getting smoked salmon from Lidgate, a very famous and usually excellent local butcher. But their smoked salmon is unspeakable. The worst ever in the history of the planet. I keep forgetting to cancel it, so they keep delivering it. As I was going to the première of Michael Caine's new film *The Prestige*, I had an apple juice at home with two small chocolate biscuits. At the première, by each seat, was a plastic bottle of Evian water – risky, I thought, as the film ran two hours and 10 minutes! Also a large bag of popcorn. I ate the popcorn! At the after-première party I had one small fishcake canapé. Night weight 78.4kg.

MONDAY 6 NOVEMBER
Morning weight 77.2kg or 12st 2¼lbs. Very good, that. Dropped a pound! Breakfast: sheep's milk yoghurt with granulated brown sugar, clementine juice. 11-ish: coffee-Scotch-chocolate-milk. At lunch trying out yet another housekeeper, a Filipino who provided the worst over-cooked duck ever. Quite a good apple crumble. Okay vegetables but the roast potatoes were second-rate. She ain't getting the job. No pm coffee! Dinner was a bit disastrous. Went to E&O in Notting Hill with Geraldine and Dinah. Had the usual edamame, two dumplings – date gyoza and prawn, spare ribs, crispy pork belly, black cod with egg rice, and mineral water. This will not look good on the scales tomorrow morning! But you have to break out occasionally. That's permitted on the Fat Pig Diet! Night weight 78kg.

TUESDAY 7 NOVEMBER
Morning weight 77.1kg or 12st 2lbs. Miracle. Down again! Some people are saying to me, 'Don't lose any more weight, you'll look scraggy!' But I've still got a stomach, albeit much, much, much smaller than it was. So onwards and downwards. Breakfast: usual sheep's milk yoghurt, brown sugar, clementine juice. 11-ish: Scotch-coffee-chocolate-milk. Lunch, prepared by my assistant Dinah: a Lidgate small steak and kidney pie (I ate two-thirds) with broccoli. Dinner: apple juice and a

few pickings by hand from yesterday's duck. One-hour walk in park. Night weight 77.3kg.

WEDNESDAY 8 NOVEMBER

Morning weight 76.5kg or 12st ¾lb. Down one and a quarter pounds. Well, I ate very little yesterday. I feel all the better for it. Breakfast: sheep's milk yoghurt, brown sugar, clementine juice. 11-ish: coffee-chocolate-Scotch-milk. Lunch at Scalini with Paola. I had some bread and butter, tiny bit of Parmesan, tagliolini with truffles, an incredibly good grilled sole with broad beans and broccoli, fresh mint tea. Dinner: just apple juice. One-hour walk. I really am being unbelievably good! Did eat four small pieces of Irish fudge during the day. It arrived in the post, who from I do not know. Then I ate three more after 'dinner'! Night weight 76.7kg.

THURSDAY 9 NOVEMBER

Morning weight 75.7kg or 11st 13lbs. Note please I am below twelve stone! I am well below the three-and-a-half-stone weight loss that is announced on the cover of this very book. This is good – it means I have some leeway. Particularly as I have to go out to dinner tonight. Breakfast: sheep's milk yoghurt, brown sugar, clementine juice. By 10.45am I'd already had three pieces of Irish fudge. It's a menace, the carton being on my desk. 11.30: half-size coffee-Scotch-chocolate-milk. That was a pathetic attempt to make up for the fudge! Lunch, a major disaster! As we had no housekeeper to try out (I've settled on the Portuguese lady who walked on me a few years ago!) Joanna Kanska, one of my assistants, accompanied me to the Papaya Tree Thai restaurant in Kensington High Street. This was recommended by my perfect neighbour, the legendary rock guitarist (Led Zeppelin, in case you're living in a cave) Jimmy Page. We had at least five main-course dishes because I wanted to try everything. The very excellent waiter, Pon Songpol, said, 'It's much too much.' We ate nearly everything with ease. We had: prawns with noodles, a mixed seafood soup with oysters and tofu, beef in a delicious sauce with chilli and basil, green chicken curry in a coconut sauce, white rice, sweet and sour pork. Then, as if that wasn't enough, we shared one dessert of mango with sticky rice and a second dessert of golden banana, which is deep-fried, topped with syrup and accompanied by a vanilla ice cream! Not a dieter's lunch. The green tea we finished with didn't make it that either. Then – it gets worse! – I had to go to dinner at Cecconi's because I was giving a birthday party for Paola. I'd promised her that since last year when she became too ill to do anything. They did a great job. Champagne followed by various appetisers including Italian sausages, mashed cod on baguette, aubergine, mozzarella and tomatoes, fried calamari, Parma ham, and pâté on toast. I also ate some bread. So I felt I'd had a full meal before some really excellent spaghetti with tomato sauce and basil appeared. The main course was wild sea bass with porcini and veggies and potatoes. Then a millefeuille birthday cake. And I ate a few biscuit petits fours as well! Later at Fifty, a very elegant club and disco in St James's, I had a couple of non-alcoholic cocktails. This has been a very heavy eating day. Night weight 77.5kg.

FRIDAY 10 NOVEMBER

Morning weight 76.7kg or 12st 1lb. A rise of two pounds in one day. That's what happens when you return to old habits. Nothing wrong in doing it occasionally, as long as you pull back the next day. But if you pig out for a week, you'll likely put on a stone (14 pounds in case you forgot!) and then you're on the road to ruin. It can happen very easily if you're not as superbly disciplined as I've become. Breakfast: sheep's milk yoghurt, brown sugar, clementine juice. 11-ish: coffee-chocolate-Scotch-milk. Lunch bought from local Luscious Organic shop by Geraldine was basmati brown rice and a vegetarian tikka masala with tofu, beans, broccoli, tomatoes, sweet peppers and other stuff. It was all disgustingly healthy. Tasted okay. It was weight-resistant. Before lunch I ate three small pieces of fudge! 4-ish: coffee-Scotch-milk. Early evening, a glass of red wine, unsalted cashew nuts and raisins. One-hour walk. Then fresh apple juice plus some water biscuit, butter and smoked salmon. Not a lot of any of this, but more than it should have been. Night weight 77.4kg.

SATURDAY 11 NOVEMBER

Morning weight 76.5kg or 12st ¾lb. Not an enormous weight loss! A quarter of a pound! So why, on the way up, before breakfast, from swimming pool to bedroom, did I stop over in the office and eat a piece of Irish fudge? Because I'm an idiot. Still, I am below my newest target weight zone of 12 stone two pounds to 12 stone five pounds. Breakfast: sheep's milk yoghurt, brown sugar, clementine juice. When you get stressed, you eat. This happened to me at noon today when I phoned Addison Lee, a well-known chauffeur car company. I'd recently set up an account with their Chairman, John Griffin. As my chauffeur, unbelievably, would rather spend the weekend with his own family than with me, I had to get a car to go to the Banqueting Hall this evening for Gordon Ramsay's 40th-birthday party. I listened to the dread recorded instructions, pressed one for account customers and gave the pick-up time, 7pm, to an operative (had to tell him the address of Whitehall twice). He took all the details, then said, 'I can't book you a car for seven. I can only do ten to seven or twenty past.' I found that amazing. I was about to say, 'Forget it and close my account' but he got in first, saying, 'I'll ask a supervisor if I can book you for seven.' Then he was gone. I was left listening to recorded music. Unbelievable! Eventually I rang off, dialled again and asked for a supervisor. Got more recorded music. This was becoming a total nightmare. The time I'd wasted was beyond belief. Any other car company, when asked for a car at seven, would give you a car at seven or say, 'We're busy, we can't do it.' Eventually I got an Addison Lee supervisor and closed the account. Then I called another company, which found sending out chauffeur cars quite a simple operation! I was so stressed at the incompetence of Addison Lee I ate seven pieces of fudge! For lunch Geraldine had done a bit of shopping. I personally grilled some pork sausages and tomatoes. I also had some smoked salmon. And fresh apple juice. Pm: one-hour walk. Dinner: Gordon Ramsay's 40th-birthday cele-bration. A couple of canapés. Lobster thermidor followed by an excellent T-bone steak with sauce béarnaise and chunky hand-cut chips. I had the waitress remove my plate before I'd scoffed the lot. Dessert was superb apple crumble and custard. Cabaret included Rory Bremner, who did his usual excellent impersonation of me, and Al Murray, the pub landlord, who had a joke on me too. Night weight 78.1kg.

SUNDAY 12 NOVEMBER

Morning weight 77.1kg or 12st 2lbs. Not surprisingly up a pound and a quarter. Breakfast: sheep's milk yoghurt, brown sugar, mix of clementine and orange juice! There's a variation for you. It's because, with no staff in on Sunday, I had to squeeze the juice myself. Who says I'm stupid in the kitchen? Lunch at the River Café. Bruschetta, Buck's Fizz, tagliolini with mushrooms, roast partridge with squash and bacon, a clementine sorbet. As usual at this restaurant, all excellent. Walk in park slightly interrupted by rain. Watched *Inside Man* in my cinema, starring Denzel Washington, Jodie Foster, Clive Owen. Pretty good. Dinner: apple juice, water biscuits, jam, butter. Night weight 78kg.

MONDAY 13 NOVEMBER

Morning weight 76.6kg or 12st ¾lb. Good weight loss, that. Onwards and downwards. Breakfast: sheep's milk yoghurt, brown sugar, clementine juice. 11-ish: coffee-chocolate-Scotch-milk-small amount of granulated brown sugar! As the new Portuguese lady housekeeper only arrived at 9.30 this morning, the chauffeur bought a steak and kidney pie and a shepherd's pie from Lidgate and the new lady did that for lunch plus cabbage, carrots and mashed swedes. 4-ish: coffee-chocolate-Scotch-milk-tiny bit of brown sugar. Alterations tailor, Michael, came again with a mass of taken-in trousers and jackets. I'd marked how much the trousers should be taken in and he said I was wrong and changed some of them to less tightening. I was right. So about six pairs had to go back yet again. I tell you, what with that and preparing the shirts for the takers-inners, it ain't easy losing weight. But it is worth it. 6pm: glass of red wine plus bowl of unsalted cashew nuts and raisins. One-hour walk followed by fresh apple juice and a small piece of water biscuit with butter. This freshly made apple juice is a delight. Am I deluding myself or do I really like it, more or less alone, for dinner? Either way I don't get hungry after that. I don't need to eat anything else. Strange for a man who'd gobble two cartons of ice cream as an after-dinner snack. It shows that when you get into the habit of dieting there is a seismic shift in what you thought was your normal, and untouchable, eating pattern. Night weight 77.1kg.

TUESDAY 14 NOVEMBER
Morning weight 76.2kg or 12st. These apple juice dinners are paying off! Breakfast as usual. 11-ish: coffee-chocolate-Scotch-milk-little brown sugar. Lunch with our new Portuguese housekeeper: brilliantly cooked sea bass, anchovy sauce, grilled tomatoes, spinach, broccoli. No question this woman knows how to cook! On her trial she did an incredible chocolate mousse. I dare not ask for that again! 4pm: coffee-chocolate-Scotch-milk-little

brown sugar. Pre-dinner, a glass of red wine and two types of smoked salmon on toothpicks! One was M&S, which Geraldine had read came top in some survey of pure, organic smoked salmon. It tasted rather salty and not very good. Then tried the local Luscious Organic smoked salmon. That was far better. Then a one-hour walk. On returning, a large glass of freshly made apple juice. What a difference there is in genuinely fresh (i.e. drunk within seconds of coming out of the mixer) apple juice to that muck you get as so-called 'fresh' in bottles or plastic containers. There's just no comparison. The really fresh stuff has warmth, softness, texture, taste. The other is ridiculous. The same applies to orange juice and any other fruit or vegetable juice. Before bed I had half a bar of Roccoco milk-free, sugar-free chocolate! Night weight 77kg.

WEDNESDAY 15 NOVEMBER
Morning weight 75.9kg or 11st 13¼lbs. Please note I am nearer four stone lighter than I used to be, rather than the three and a half stone advertised on this book cover! Breakfast: sheep's milk yoghurt, brown sugar, clementine juice. Lunch: roast chicken, two small roast potatoes, parsnips, carrots, beans. 4-ish: coffee-chocolate-Scotch-milk-brown sugar. Unbelievable letter arrives by fax from John Griffin, Chairman of Addison Lee plc car rental. He seems to think holding on for almost four minutes (minus four seconds), listening to dreary recorded music, whilst waiting for one of his operatives is nothing to complain about. And he makes the utterly bizarre statement: 'Most of Whitehall looks like it could be the Banqueting Hall.'

The Whitehall I know has a theatre, apartment buildings
– mainly Victorian – and rows of shops, including trinket
shops and cafés. How most of that looks like one of the
most famous 17th-century landmarks of London I do not
know. I hope Mr Griffin's drivers know London better
than he does! For dinner I was on my own as Geraldine
had gone to see her family in Paris. I had some Marks &
Spencer organic smoked salmon (pretty good) and some
freshly made apple juice (wonderful). Then, feeling
peckish, I had 100 grams of Beluga caviar on some
unbuttered water biscuit. At restaurant prices that's
about £400 worth. Long as it doesn't put on weight, who
cares! Night weight 76.9kg.

THURSDAY 16 NOVEMBER
Morning weight 75.9kg or 11st 13¼lbs. No rise, no fall.
I'm getting worried about my shirts! I've had them taken
in to a body measurement of 48 inches, sometimes 49
inches. That's around stomach etc. Even at this low
weight it's looking a bit iffy, possibly tight. I must ask
opinions today. These are the problems that come when
you lose over six inches on your waist! Breakfast: sheep's
milk yoghurt, four teaspoonfuls of brown granulated
sugar, clementine juice. I really like this breakfast! Mind
you, before dieting I usually had just slices of orange or
grapefruit. Probably even less fattening. 11-ish: Scotch-
milk-coffee-chocolate-brown sugar. Lunch: grilled sole,
spinach, beans, parsnips. 4-ish: coffee-Scotch-milk-
chocolate-brown sugar. Dinner at The Wolseley, next to
an acquaintance, the brilliant Mel Brooks, with his son
who is an author. I had not one, but two vanilla

milkshakes – one to start and one to end. In between a bit of bread and butter, smoked salmon, cabbage, spinach, mashed potato. Not an ideally slimming meal. But we dieters have to let rip occasionally. Early to bed (before 9pm) with a Rohypnol, also known as the date rape pill. A wonderful sleeping pill. I wanted to be sure to be fresh and vibrant (hah! hah!) as I'm shooting some more commercials for esure car insurance tomorrow at a shopping mall in Croydon. Just to get to Croydon you need to be well rested. What a ghastly journey I see from checking my map. Night weight 76.9kg.

FRIDAY 17 NOVEMBER
Morning weight 76.1kg or 11st 13¾lbs. Well, you don't have two milkshakes in the evening without putting on a bit! Breakfast: sheep's milk yoghurt, brown sugar, clementine juice. As I was being made up at home: coffee-Scotch-milk-sugar-chocolate. Then a one-hour drive to the Centrale shopping mall in Croydon! That's where I was to 'act' in the esure commercials. I drank a lot of hot water with lemon and honey, which is good for my voice. I lunched with Peter Wood, the Chairman of esure, in a House of Fraser store in the mall. I had a 'chicken vegetable udon noodle soup', which was horrific. Didn't consume much of it. Then I took some noodles from the adjacent sushi bar as they travelled round on the counter. Followed by, from the restaurant menu, a chicken teriyaki. This was similar to the soup! Only much better. Basically just chicken and noodles. Finished off with apple pie and cream. In the afternoon, to keep the energy level up, my assistant Dinah got a

selection of jelly babies and fried egg sweets and one mini Mars bar from the film company. I ate too many of the sweets. At home for dinner (an hour-and-a-half drive back because it was pouring with rain!) I had 100 grams of Beluga caviar on some water biscuits, apple juice and one chocolate biscuit. Night weight 77kg.

SATURDAY 18 NOVEMBER

Morning weight 76.4kg or 12st ½lb. It's odd – normally I lose one kilogram during the night. Last night I only lost 0.6kg! I'm three-quarters of a pound up, so I'd better take it off. Breakfast: sheep's milk yoghurt, back to jam with it, clementine juice. 10-ish: coffee-milk-chocolate-Scotch. Lunch at The Wolseley with Paola. My literary agent, Ed Victor, and Mel Brooks were at the next table. I had lamb shank (delicious), a vanilla milkshake (very piggy of me), mashed potatoes and apple crumble with custard. And a taste of Paola's biscuit selection. Then we went on to see St Alban, the new restaurant of Jeremy King and Chris Corbin, ex-bosses of The Ivy, Le Caprice and J Sheekey, current owners of The Wolseley. St Alban was still boarded up, but they were trying it out for friends. Was knocked out with how elegant it was. Very 1950s. Had a chat with Charles Saatchi (he needs this book, bless him – has he put on weight!) and Nigella Lawson, but only consumed a limoncello. Back home, alone, as Geraldine was still in Paris. Dinner was just apple juice plus one small chocolate biscuit. Night weight 77.2kg.

SUNDAY 19 NOVEMBER

Morning weight 76.5kg or 12st ¾lb. I really don't see why I put on a quarter of a pound when all I had for dinner was apple juice and a small chocolate biscuit! Maybe it's because, with Geraldine in Paris, I'm not forced to take a one-hour evening walk. She's back this morning, so I'll walk today. Breakfast: mix of clementine and orange juice, sheep's milk yoghurt, brown granulated sugar. Lunch at St Alban. I had bruschetta of Monte Enebro goat's cheese and cherry tomatoes. Then slow-roasted black pig with turnip tops on a base of pumpkin. Jeremy King tells me the pig is from Spain and fed on hazelnuts and walnuts! Tried a bit of bread and breadsticks. No butter. For dessert, pistachio ice cream with zabaglione affogato. It was all great, except for some strange Portuguese still mineral water that was awful beyond belief. Then walked for an hour in St James's Park and Whitehall. Saw *United 93* in my private cinema. About one of the hijacked planes on 9/11. Bloody good! Dinner: glass of apple juice, one small chocolate biscuit. Night weight 77.1kg.

MONDAY 20 NOVEMBER

Morning weight 76.1kg or 11st 13¾lbs. Back under 12 stone. That's always nice! Breakfast: clementine juice, sheep's milk yoghurt with jam. 11-ish: single malt Scotch-milk-coffee-sugar-chocolate. Lunch: very good veal chop, cabbage, beans, ratatouille. Housekeeper asked for a sofa bed because her daughter is coming over for Christmas. I said, 'We'll get you a blow-up mattress for the floor.' I'm all heart. At least she thinks she'll still be here at Christmas. Last time I employed her she walked after a week! Evening food started with two glasses of champagne and fresh orange juice accompanied by smoked salmon on toothpicks and little bits of water biscuits and butter. Then Geraldine and I took an hour-long walk in the park. On returning I had a plate of smoked salmon with lemon and a glass of apple juice. Night weight 76.6kg.

TUESDAY 21 NOVEMBER
Morning weight 75.7kg or 11st 13lbs. Almost a triumph! It really does show that if you keep the evening food intake seriously down, you're ahead of the game. Breakfast: clementine juice, sheep's milk yoghurt, jam. 11-ish: Scotch-coffee-chocolate-milk-sugar. Kara from Watlington had, unusually, made a mess of some curtains and blinds for me. She came to re-measure and brought me some unbelievably good vanilla cookies she had made herself! 'If you ever get out of curtains, you can always open a cake shop!' I advised, before going off to lunch at Fifty, a gambling club in St James's with great restaurant, bars and disco. This was for the Old Vic Theatre, hosted by Robert Earl. Elton John was there, plus Kevin Spacey and other stars. At drinks beforehand a very famous actor and his famous wife went on at great length about how ghastly J Sheekey had become and how awful the service was and so on. They didn't realise, until I introduced him, that the man they were talking to was Richard Caring, the owner of J Sheekey! I had smoked salmon and lobster, then roast beef and Yorkshire pud with roast potatoes and veg. Left a lot of it even though it was good. I departed

after the auction and before the bread and butter pudding. A man on a diet shouldn't stay for bread and butter pudding! Dinner: first a Buck's Fizz at home (that's champagne and orange juice), then in my kitchen some home-made minestrone soup with grated Parmesan, three water biscuits with butter, one small chocolate biscuit. Then I attacked the vanilla cookies left by my curtain lady and finished them off. You see, there's no such thing as a reformed pig. Once a pig always a pig. At least I admit it! Night weight 76.6kg.

WEDNESDAY 22 NOVEMBER
Morning weight 75.7kg or 11st 13lbs. Miracle those cookies didn't do damage. Maybe it'll turn up tomorrow. Breakfast: sheep's milk yoghurt, jam, clementine juice. 11-ish: Scotch-coffee-chocolate-milk-sugar. Lunch: halibut (rather a heavy fish, didn't eat much!), fennel, broccoli, carrots, beans, béarnaise sauce. Dinner: four chocolate biscuits, apple juice. Night weight 76.1kg.

THURSDAY 23 NOVEMBER
Morning weight 75.3kg or 11st 12lbs. I'm two pounds off being four stone less than I used to be. A couple of pounds more wouldn't hurt. Give me leeway if I put on too much at Sandy Lane in Barbados, to which I go next month. 11-ish: Scotch-chocolate-coffee-milk-sugar. Lunch: a grilled poussin, two roast potatoes, mushrooms and what I think they used to call a 'bouquet' of vegetables. 4-ish: Scotch-coffee-chocolate-milk-sugar. 5.20pm: bit of chocolate cake with icing, which was my chauffeur Jim's birthday cake. Shouldn't have done that really. Still find it difficult

to resist temptation! 'You stupid, moronic pig, Winner!' That's telling me! Then with Geraldine, her son Fabrice and Dinah I had two Buck's Fizz and some handfuls of salted cashew nuts and raisins. Then went for a walk. Returned and had the juice of half an orange. Plus a further small piece of Jim's chocolate cake. Then (mistake this) I saw some superb cheeses in the fridge. So I had some Camembert and blue cheese on about eight water biscuits. Night weight 75.6kg.

FRIDAY 24 NOVEMBER
Morning weight 74.8kg or 11st 11lbs. I am one pound off being not three and a half stone lighter, but four stone lighter! Will I vanish altogether? I hope not. It would make too many people happy. Breakfast: clementine juice, sheep's milk yoghurt with jam. 11-ish: coffee-chocolate-Scotch-milk-sugar. Lunch: grilled salmon, peas, cabbage, carrots, broccoli. I don't know if my stomach's shrunk (I guess it must have, nearly everything else has!) because I couldn't eat all the salmon. When you see a diet really succeeding you become possessed (or better put, absolutely determined) not to put on weight again. Particularly after such a public diet. And also because you feel so much better. In the afternoon the *Evening Standard* architectural writer rang me to say my local Odeon, which I'd campaigned to have saved, had not been saved but the developers were going to keep the 1935 façade. Half a victory. The developers had told the journalist I'd still have the right to take pick 'n' mix sweets from the plastic containers without charge! This goes back to when I dived in and took some before going

into a movie and ate them straight from the containers. The next day I sent the Odeon manager £100 to cover the few I'd taken and some future ones. He sent the cheque back, saying I could have sweets free whenever I wanted and also enclosed 10 free cinema seats. So I sent a cheque for £500 in the name of Odeon cinemas to the Variety Club of Great Britain, which keeps homes for crippled children. When the *Standard* journalist told me my sweet concession would be continued I said, 'That's the first bribe I'll accept!' Dinner: apple juice, cheese and water biscuits, no butter. One-hour walk. Returned to watch *Little Miss Sunshine* in my cinema. Brilliant. Then something odd! About eight years ago I chucked out my projectors and put in projection DVD and video. Where the projection room had been at the back I made a bar with a display of bottles, glasses and an enormous air-conditioning unit. But no drink had ever been drunk there. After *Little Miss Sunshine* I opened a bottle of Bols peppermint liqueur that had sat on the glass shelf for eight years. Geraldine got some ice from the machine in the next room. We had the iced peppermint liqueur. Then I opened a small can of R White's lemonade from the bar icebox and added some more peppermint drink. Very nice. Then I went to bed. Night weight 75.3kg.

SATURDAY 25 NOVEMER

Morning weight 74.4kg or 11st 10lbs. I'm now four stone lighter than I used to be! That's 56 pounds! Or 25 kilograms. A lot of fat has fled! When I started this diary on 6 May, exactly 29 weeks ago, I was 12 stone 12 pounds. The idea was to show how to stay at an acceptably low weight. But I've shed a further one stone two pounds! On a 'holding' diet. I hope you're learning! Breakfast: sheep's milk yoghurt, jam, clementine juice. 11-ish: coffee-chocolate-Scotch-milk-sugar. Lunch at The Ivy: Buck's Fizz, then their set menu – endive, pear and walnut salad, braised beef with carrots, mashed potatoes (added butter), gravy, some bread and butter. In the old days I'd have eaten all the two chunks of braised beef. Now I couldn't. Maybe my stomach has shrunk inwardly as well as outwardly? Finished with vanilla pannacotta and rhubarb. In the afternoon went for a walk with Geraldine, which diverted to an enormous Tesco store. I don't do shopping. But as Geraldine picked a few things I grabbed a packet of plantain crisps and ate them. Paid for them, of course. They were ghastly. I definitely shouldn't shop for myself. At home had some apple juice with a little cheese and water biscuits. Watched *Friends with Money* in my private cinema. Very good. Then again had Bols peppermint liqueur with R White's lemonade and ice at the cinema bar. Around midnight took one chocolate, which was sitting by my bedroom kitchenette basin, plus one cup of hot chocolate and Horlicks mixed, no sugar. Night weight 75.5kg.

SUNDAY 26 NOVEMBER

Morning weight 74.7kg or 11st 10¾lbs. Don't know why I put on three-quarters of a pound yesterday. Breakfast: sheep's milk yoghurt, jam, clementine juice. Lunch at Michael Caine's country house. Before lunch I ate some nuts. Dining were six women, Michael and me. As usual the food was superb beyond belief. This was Michael's Thanksgiving Day meal – turkey, marvellous sausages, roast potatoes as only he can do them, mixed veg, parsnips, gravy. Dessert was bread and butter pudding, plums in mascarpone and Häagen-Dazs ice cream. I also had a few after-dinner mints. 'Don't lose any more weight,' said Michael. I assured him with what he'd given me to eat I certainly wouldn't lose any today! Dinner: apple juice, 200 grams of Beluga caviar on matzos. No butter. One-hour walk. Then watched a strange film, *Running with Scissors*. Bizarre but memorable. Just before bed – foolishly – a piece of buttered toast with Marmite. Geraldine, rightly, groaned yet again at my ongoing weaknesses. Night weight 76kg.

MONDAY 27 NOVEMBER
Morning weight 75.5kg or 11st 12½lbs. Shows how diet-disaster is always around the corner. There I was, crowing, two days ago, that I was 11 stone 10 pounds, and four stone lighter, and here I am up two and a half pounds. I'm afraid perpetual vigilance is required unless I want to find myself a fat pig again! Breakfast: sheep's milk yoghurt with brown sugar, clementine juice. 11-ish: coffee-Scotch-chocolate-milk-sugar. I phoned Jeremy King, co-owner of The Wolseley, to book for lunch. Jeremy seemed a bit irked. I'd told a story in the *Sunday Times* about how, for his last day with partner Chris Corbin at The Ivy, I'd made a reservation as I was intending to make a farewell speech for Chris and Jeremy. Jeremy personally took the booking. He was still the boss. And for the first time ever he gave me a piece

of paper to confirm it. The day before I was due to show up the general manager, Mitchell Everard, now with Jeremy at St Alban, rang and said, 'You can't have your usual table. Mr Scott's there.' In the *Sunday Times* I wrote: 'Anyway, I didn't go. I'm not prepared to be messed about by staff.' That was after giving St Alban a rave. Jeremy said, 'What you wrote about the booking wasn't true.' 'You know it was true, Jeremy. You personally handed me the reservation slip!' I said in amazement. 'But it didn't mention the table,' said Jeremy. 'Where did you think I was going to sit? On the toilet?' I responded. 'I've sat at the same table in The Ivy for every booking forever.' 'It didn't make you look good,' said Jeremy. 'People might think badly of you.' 'I haven't given a shit what people think about me for 50 years. I'm certainly not starting now!' I said, laughing. Jeremy is quite simply London's best restaurateur and has been – along with his partner Chris Corbin – for ages. At The Wolseley I had some roll and butter, salad niçoise, grilled plaice, a vanilla milkshake, mint tea. Dinner at home: minestrone soup. One-hour walk. Even paid my congestion charge for today on the phone. Very proud I managed that! Night weight 76.4kg.

TUESDAY 28 NOVEMBER

Morning weight 75.2kg or 11st 11¾lbs. A tiny drop. Whoopee! Breakfast: sheep's milk yoghurt, jam, clementine juice. As Geraldine was in Paris seeing her family before we go away for Christmas, for lunch I went back to St Alban, with Paola. I had some excellent bread, a Buck's Fizz, fried calamari, a very good rabbit stew with mashed potatoes and lentils, and finished off with vanilla pannacotta and fresh mint tea. St Alban is still on try-outs at half price. They don't let it get full. A friend of mine phoned to book for dinner on Thursday and was told, 'You have to come before six or after ten.' I think he was angling for me to intrude. But if that's what King and Corbin want, far be it from me to interfere. For dinner I just had chicken soup and smoked salmon. Night weight 76.4kg.

WEDNESDAY 29 NOVEMBER

Morning weight 75.9kg or 11st 13 ¼lbs. That's really odd! One and a half pounds up after a light eating day. And I only went down 0.5kg overnight when normally I go down a kilogram! But that's dieting life! Full of mystery. Breakfast: sheep's milk yoghurt, jam, clementine juice. 11-ish: coffee-chocolate-Scotch-milk-sugar. Lunch at home: rack of lamb, leeks in a sauce, mixed vegetables. Just after lunch over 2,000 of my Christmas cards arrived. All have to be signed by hand and many hand-written messages added to them! Made a major start. I guess we posted over 250 and got another 250 ready to be posted first thing in the morning! 4-ish: coffee-chocolate-Scotch-milk-sugar. Dinner: apple juice, then water biscuits, cheese, a little jam, rather a lot of strawberries! After dinner sat signing Christmas cards and watched *I'm a Celebrity, Get Me Out of Here*! Very good programme! Love to see nonentities under stress! David Gest is the funniest person I've seen on TV for years. His routine about an albino hotel that's all black, called Albino Heights in Detroit, was absolute magic. The other lightweight so-called celebrities didn't know whether to believe him or not! He went in hated by everyone. He's coming out brilliantly. I've voted for him to stay about 40 times! Night weight 76.8kg.

THURSDAY 30 NOVEMBER

Morning weight 75.7kg or 11st 13lbs. Breakfast: clementine juice, sheep's milk yoghurt, brown sugar. 11-ish: coffee-Scotch-chocolate-milk-sugar. Lunch at The Wolseley with Paola. First I had almost two sorts of incredible cake things they give at the bar with drinks. Then chopped liver, then herring in cream. Dessert was a vanilla milkshake and some biscuits followed by mint tea. In the early evening a computer company took over my laptop by remote control to install a new Norton virus-protection device. It wasn't completed for some reason. Next thing my computer crashed. This book was not saved on disk. It vanished. I was in total panic! Went to dinner at St Alban and had some bread, ham, a shrimp salad and orange sorbet. All sensational. A lady came up and greeted me. I had no idea who she was. She went to sit nearby with another woman. I went over. 'What's your name?' I asked. She said, 'You should know. I slept with you for a year!' Turns out she's an ex-girlfriend for whom I had and still have particularly warm feelings. The lady she was with is her daughter, who works for King and Corbin (who own St Alban as H and R, whatever that means). Night weight 76.6kg.

FRIDAY 1 DECEMBER

Morning weight 75.6kg or 11st 12¾lbs. Breakfast: clementine juice, sheep's milk yoghurt, jam. 11-ish: coffee-chocolate-milk-sugar-Scotch. Finished signing all the Christmas cards, including 500 to bookshop managers! Lunch: grilled sole, beans, broccoli, carrots. 4-ish: coffee-chocolate-sugar-Scotch-milk. 6.30pm: apple juice and quite a few strawberries. One-hour walk in park. A small amount of Rococo dairy-free and sugar-free chocolate. Ken, in Newcastle, dealt partly with my laptop problems, which were horrific. The cursor kept turning into an egg timer! We uninstalled the Norton AntiVirus and Ken will come over at the weekend with a simpler version. I hate computers, laptops, radios with more than two buttons, remote controls for anything, and telephones that dance, go shopping, take photos and tell you how to behave. I hate everything electronic except simple light bulbs. And I'm furious because last night, when I wasn't here to vote, they threw David Gest off *I'm a Celebrity, Get Me Out of Here*. As you can see, my life is full of meaningful things. Long may it so continue. Night weight 76.5kg,

SATURDAY 2 DECEMBER

Morning weight 75.5kg or 11st 12½lbs. Breakfast: sheep's milk yoghurt, jam, clementine juice. Ken came to fix my laptop after it had been 'contaminated' by the Norton AntiVirus. He'd had one hour's sleep in Newcastle! I made him a coffee personally and a smoked salmon sandwich. Lunch for me was at San Lorenzo: started with orange juice, then salami, raw baby artichoke shavings, mozzarella, tomato, rocket, avocado, then spaghetti with tomato sauce, then chocolate ice cream (theirs is the best!) and then an espresso coffee with, foolishly, five chocolate macaroons. One-hour walk in park. Dinner: apple juice, matzos, butter and jam. Watched *Pirates of the Caribbean, Dead Man's Chest* in my private cinema. Very entertaining. Afterwards had a Bols peppermint liqueur with ice and White's lemonade. Found that water was coming in under the bar sink. Luckily I have a tin tray there to stop the water seeping anywhere else. Need a plumber! Night weight 76.4kg.

SUNDAY 3 DECEMBER

Morning weight 75.6kg or 11st 12¾lbs. Keeping my end down. Breakfast: orange juice (orange, not clementine, because on Sunday I have to squeeze the fruit myself), jam, sheep's milk yoghurt. I've changed newsagents. The first one went after seven years because he didn't deliver the *Sunday Times* when asked to. Next one went after four weeks because last week the papers were soaking wet. Today, first delivery from a new one – and the Culture section of the *Sunday Times* had a big damp patch through half of it! How? The papers were totally encased in a black plastic rubbish sack and tied up with string! I dried it with a hairdryer before passing it to Geraldine, who reads such things. Lunch at the River Café: prosecco with pomegranate juice, bruschetta, followed by tagliolini with truffles (an amazing £69 plus service!), then partridge with beans and chard. Dessert was a chocolate and chestnut sorbet, which was so rich it tasted very much like ice cream to me. One-hour walk.

Dinner: apple juice, matzos, butter, cheese. Watched the film *Infamous*, about Truman Capote, in my private cinema. Very good and touching. Night weight 76.8kg.

MONDAY 4 DECEMBER
Morning weight 75.9kg or 11st 13¼lbs. Hmmm. Up half a pound! Cheated this morning and took a Frumil tablet. This reduces water in the body. I used to take one about once a month. I've got a tiny cold. They sometimes help. Breakfast (this'll really not surprise you!): clementine juice, sheep's milk yoghurt, jam. Lunch with Paola at The Wolseley (she's having even more problems with her health and had yet again been visiting Harley Street). There was my current hero, David Gest, fresh from his triumphs in *I'm a Celebrity, Get Me Out of Here*. He told me he'd now got his own TV show from it. I said I'd known that it would happen soon as I saw how funny he was. Good luck to him. I ate chopped liver, herring, too many sweet biscuits and a vanilla milkshake. Before one-hour walk, two Buck's Fizz at home. Dinner: apple juice, matzos, butter, cheese, pickle. Modest amount! Night weight 75.1kg.

TUESDAY 5 DECEMBER
Morning weight 74kg or 11st 9lbs. This is one pound over four stone I've lost! Slightly distorted because I took a Frumil water-loss pill yesterday as I had phlegmy cough. This is our last day of record for a seven-month diet. So it will be no surprise to you to know breakfast consisted of sheep's milk yoghurt, jam and clementine juice, and 11-ish I had coffee-Scotch-chocolate-milk-sugar. Lunch: a

poussin, roast potatoes, mixed veggies. 4pm-ish: the usual Scotch-coffee-chocolate-milk-sugar. Dinner at E&O in Notting Hill: edamame, date gyozas, prawn dumplings, baby spare ribs, pork belly, black cod, egg rice, veg, mixed sorbets. Night weight 75.9kg.

The next morning, now outside our seven-month diet diary, I was 74.8kg or 11st 11lbs. So I was one pound under being four stone lighter than I used to be. If that's not (a) a triumph and (b) a miracle, I don't know what is. Actually it's mind over food-matter, discipline where once there was abandonment, sense where once was idiocy. You too can do it. I am thinner, happier, fitter, lovelier and all round better. Why deny that for yourself? My new target weight – note it's diminished as the weeks have gone by – is now between 11 stone 12 pounds and 12 stone two pounds.

But now I face the biggest test ever since I started fairly serious dieting. In under two weeks I fly to the Sandy Lane Hotel, Barbados. Home of the most tempting buffets. All full of fattening things. I can't sit in the suite and make an apple juice as I've been doing at home. During the day I'll be tempted by banana daiquiris, pina coladas, fruit punches and all things sweet and fat-providing. How will I fare after three weeks there? Will I be back on the road to ruin? Will I be the miserable possessor of hundreds of jackets, trousers and shirts I can no longer get into? Will I be able to pull back? How much damage will I have to pull back from? How can I go out promoting this diet book looking fat and flaccid? I'm panicking. On my return from Barbados, I will reveal all. Thanks for hanging on this far.

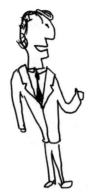

AND I'M STILL
ONLY 12 STONE!

Chapter Six

Postscript

Oh boy, did things turn out differently from what I'd expected! I arrived at Sandy Lane on 16 December, a cheery idiot, determined to stay slim. Through the following days I did put on a bit of weight. On 31 December, the last day of fairly normal life, I was 12 stone two pounds. Still three and a half stone lighter than I had been. I wasn't feeling terribly well on New Year's Eve, but I went down for the buffet dinner, although Geraldine reminds me I hardly left the table and went to bed soon after midnight. On 1 January I started to shake. I assumed it was something that would pass by.

It did not. As you know from the beginning of this book, I had contracted Vibrio Vulnificus, a disease so rare that no one knew about it. After 19 operations and five and a half months in hospital, I survived! My weight went down from 12 stone 2 pounds on 1 January in Barbados to eleven stone. I have now gone up to 11 stone 12 pounds, which is where I'd like to stay. (In case you're concerned, my catching VV had nothing whatsoever to do with my diet!) I can no longer do as much exercise as I used to because in debriding my leg (that's hacking away bits that kept rotting!), the surgeon had to hack off my Achilles tendon. I won't go into a major description of what happened thereafter. It might spoil your Christmas lunch. Or indeed your intake of any food at all! Now, more than ever, I am having to follow my own dieting dictum – EAT LESS. And I'm achieving it. After all, I can't appear to plug this book looking like the fat slob I was at 15 stone 10 pounds.

Other than 'eat less', I'd like to pass on some personal advice to you, which you may think eccentric. Never – and I do mean never – eat raw fish of any kind from anywhere. This VV thing that nearly did me in is getting less and less rare. There are now cases in Europe from oysters not farmed or picked from warm seas. It is my personal view that all our rivers and seas are now so polluted, it's not worth taking the risk, however small, that you may end up with this dreadful killer illness. It consumed well over seven months of my life. I was within a millimetre of death five times.

I don't want to end on a down note. You are well and I want you to stay well. I want you to be reasonably slim, happy and self-confident. I've no doubt at all that if you follow the dieting advice in this book you will achieve all those things. So only eat half the scoop of ice cream. Take a few bites of the bread roll and leave the rest. Keep eating whatever taste gives you the most pleasure. But learn to leave a lot of it. If you're out to dinner and your hostess thinks you're insulting her cooking by not stuffing yourself solid, so what? You have your own life and well-being to protect.

I do hope you'll have the strength of purpose to use my diet as a guide for you. Either way – whether you say, 'Winner be damned, I will have that enormous plate of ice cream' or you say, 'If a fat pig like Winner could do it, so can I' – I wish you well. Be happy. Enjoy life. But show discipline!

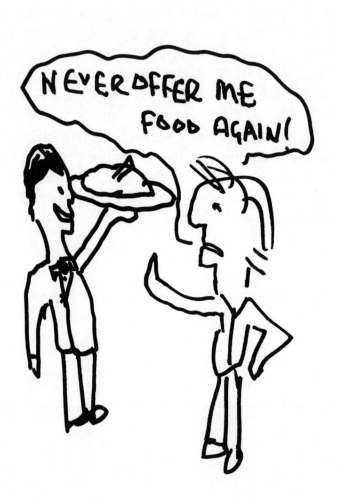